The Fibro Bible

*Discover the Science of Gut Flora, Gasotransmitters, and
Tensegrity for Eliminating Fibromyalgia and Chronic Fatigue*

By

Andrew Miles, DOM & Xuelan Qiu, PhD

ISBN- 978-15333138-2-9

Dedication

This book is dedicated to your trillions of nerves currently disintegrating under the pressures of fibromyalgia. Relief is here.

Disclaimer

This book is not intended as a substitute for the medical advice of physicians. Readers should regularly consult a physician in matters relating to their health, particularly with respect to any symptoms that might require diagnosis or medical attention. Enjoy.

Table of Contents

Foreword

DESTRUCTION THROUGHOUT

When your gut loses balance, 100 trillion microbes which were once beneficial citizens of your internal world begin to riot. They begin feasting on your intestines like a horde of microscopic zombies. This feeding causes intestinal lesions which have been associated with a host of chronic diseases such as:

Inflammatory bowel disease (IBD): An autoimmune disorder that takes the forms of Crohn's disease and ulcerative colitis.

Rheumatoid arthritis (RA): RA is an autoimmune disease that often results in bilateral inflammation of the joints.

Fungal infections: This includes everything from toenail fungus to yeast infections.

Hormonal imbalance: Hormone balance influences gut balance and gut balance influences the hypothalamic pituitary adrenal (HPA) axis, playing a role in depression, insomnia, bipolar disorder, gynecological disorders, and chronic fatigue.

Schizophrenia: Characterized by a loss of contact with reality, hallucinations, false beliefs, disorganized speech and behavior, restricted range of emotions, and impaired reasoning and problem solving; results in occupational and social dysfunction.

Obesity: Excess body weight, defined as a body mass index (BMI) of $\geq$ 30. [1] Complications include cardiovascular disorders (particularly in people with excess abdominal fat), diabetes mellitus, certain cancers, gall stones, fatty liver, cirrhosis, osteoarthritis, reproductive disorders in men and women, psychological disorders, and, for people with BMI $\geq$ 35, premature death. Obesity itself is also associated with a host of chronic diseases. It doesn't just hurt people physically; it also comes with significant financial, social, and emotional costs.

---

[1] *BMI is an easy calculation for looking at obesity among populations of people. It doesn't differentiate between fat and muscle so it's inaccurate for calculating body fat in an individual.*

Fibromyalgia: Associated with fatigue, generalized pain and sensitivity to pressure, this disease is heavily correlated with chronic fatigue, depression and anxiety.

What is fibromyalgia?

Fibromyalgia is characterized by systemic musculoskeletal pain associated with sensitive pressure points. It is often accompanied by fatigue, sleep disorders, memory challenges, and emotional distress. It is associated with a poor distribution of nitric oxide. This gives it a common etiology with multiple chemical sensitivity, chronic fatigue syndrome, and major depression, and anxiety. Approximately 3.4% of women in the United States suffer from fibromyalgia.

Women are much more likely to develop fibromyalgia than are men. Many people who have fibromyalgia also have tension headaches, temporomandibular joint (TMJ) disorders, irritable bowel syndrome as well as food sensitivities associated with gut dysbiosis.

COSTS OF FYBROMYOGIA

Direct costs for people with fibromyalgia were around

3,939 dollars per year in 2011. People with severe fibromyalgia (65.5%) spend upwards of 10,000 dollars per year. Indirect costs such as job restriction can cost 30,000 per year. Tragically, it is exactly the advice given by medical professionals that keeps people in state of permanent suffering and financial loss.

What causes Fibromyalgia?

Fibromyalgia is caused by long term stress, poor diet, and irregular sleep cycles. This creates a combination of gut dysbiosis (poor gut flora balance) improper distribution of gasotransmitters such as nitric oxide, and hormonal imbalances leading to chronic inflammation. It is a very similar etiology as chronic fatigue syndrome, multiple chemical sensitivity, and PTSD.

According to the Merk Manual:

"Fibromyalgia is a common nonarticular disorder of unknown cause characterized by generalized aching (sometimes severe); widespread tenderness of muscles, areas around tendon insertions,

and adjacent soft tissues; muscle stiffness; fatigue; and poor sleep. Diagnosis is clinical. Treatment includes exercise, local heat, stress management, drugs to improve sleep, and analgesics."

Fibromyalgia diagnosis is relatively subjective and is determined more by ruling out other diseases such as rheumatoid arthritis. There is a blood test called FM/a that identifies markers produced by immune system blood cells in people with fibromyalgia.

Fibromyalgia is often treated as a no man's land of diagnosis. Because of this, many people who have fatigue and tender points don't really have fibromyalgia at all. Some of these symptoms are rare signs of unrelated diseases that eventually present with some of the same symptoms as fibromyalgia. Some cardiac conditions can result in fatigue and tender points. To know what is and isn't' actual fibromyalgia, it's essential to see the entire picture. To do this, we will move from the dark ages of fibromyalgia superstition where the etiology is guessed upon into the light of identifying many the overlapping pathologies that go into understanding what fibromyalgia is and how to effectively treat it. The answer to fibromyalgia requires a multidisciplinary approach that looks at the body as a systemic whole.

BLIND MEN TOUCH THE ELEPHANT

A king in India once settled a debate by asking several blind men to touch an elephant. The king asked the blind men to describe what they were feeling and how it would best be used. One man grabbed the tail and said, "It is a rope. It is best used for construction projects." Another man grabbed hold of an ear and said, "It is a fan, best used for cooling the room." The third man touched the foot and said, "It is a pillar, ideal for supporting the roof." The last man touched the tusk and said, "This plow is perfect for tilling the fields."

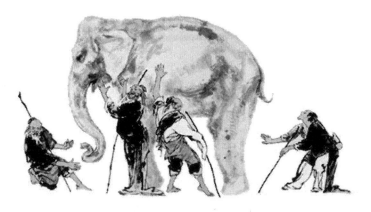

Nowadays, someone notices a trigger point associated

with fibromyalgia and assumes that fibro is completely about trigger points. Another notices pain increased with bad weather and assumes that it's all about immune factors. Another treats the thyroid and still another works through the gut flora and claims that all fibromyalgia is due to leaky gut. All of them are helpful, but still blind men groping around in the dark.

You can't discover the truth about fibromyalgia from blind isolation; you must look for it in the light of context.

THE EIGHT MAIN CAUSES OF FIBROMYALGIA

Fibromyalgia is chronic pain caused by eight separate, yet overlapping causes. The predominant factor that causes pain can and does change based on weather patterns, diet, psychological triggering, sleep, and mitochondrial levels. This variability is why fibromyalgia seems so random. For anyone who has been on a fibro forum or talked to a fibro support group, you have heard stories that are terrifying and make the situation seem bleak.

A woman is diligently practicing yoga. She is feeling better by the day and then suddenly, for no apparent reason the pain is back with a vengeance. She was doing everything "right". She summoned every bit of will power. Why was the yoga suddenly not helping anymore? This lack of understanding is terrifying and leads many to believe that they are cursed or that the situation is hopeless.

A doctor cured several patients with a special diet. It worked exceptionally for some, but not at all for others. Why?

A body worker made one person feel normal again, but caused the next patient to have an extreme spike in pain. Why?

The simple answer is because there are eight different overlapping causes. Seeing them with clarity will allow you to flexibly adapt. It will help you know what to use to help alleviate pain, when to use it, and when to stop.

In most cases all of these mechanisms are at work to a

varying degree, but one will play a predominant role and alleviating it will allow the others to follow. Finding that first domino creates a metabolic cascade that increases energy, decreases pain, and improves quality of life.

TYPE ONE: IMMUNE HYPERSENSITIVITY

Big Picture:

Imagine having the flu. The aches and pains follow a similar pattern due to the generalized immune response. Imagine the complete loss of energy, stiff neck, mental fogginess and lethargy. This is essentially what is happening with this cause of fibromyalgia.

Stiff neck and/or frozen shoulder, swollen lymphatic tissue, weak immune system, chronic inflammation associated with rhinitis, tiredness, aches, and chills.

The pain itself comes when the immune system perceives a pathogen. It responds with increased inflammatory cytokines, nitric oxide, and homocysteine levels. The increased nitric oxide around the areas of inflammation can cause muscle contraction similar to the way you might get a stiff neck when getting a common cold. This muscle tension further limits lymphatic drainage. The restricted lymphatic drainage can contribute to challenges with water retention and sweating. When this happens you will see either an absence of sweating or sweating along the back of the neck. This particular type of fibromyalgia pain wanders from place to place as the non-specific immunity tries to respond nonspecifically to the pathogen.

When this mechanism plays a predominant role in the development of fibromyalgia, people experience pain that changes with the seasons and may be worse during allergy or cold seasons. The pain tends to linger in the joints and upper back.

Key Signs:

- Stiff neck and/or frozen shoulder
- Swollen lymphatic tissue
- Chills
- Aches
- Tiredness

Treatment Strategy:

Induce sweating and stay warm. People with this kind of pain benefit from saunas and immune therapies. Lymph drainage massage has also been shown to be helpful in these cases.

As an underlying strategy we use plant-based therapies shown to regulate nitric oxide and water metabolism. To really alleviate the pain from this stage, it is essential to activate microphages and regulate T cells, B cells, and NK cells. Antiviral, antibacterial and antifungal interventions may all be used so long as they don't cause major distress to gut microbiota. It is also important during this stage to regulate bowel movements and protect the liver and the CNS.

TYPE TWO: GUT DYSBIOSIS

Poor gut balance leads to systemic inflammation causing fatigue and pain symptoms. Poor cultivation of gut flora interferes with the manufacture of vitamins, processing of amino acids, and is associated with intestinal lesions and inappropriate immune reactions. It is similar to type one, except that the cause is primarily dietary, rather than caused by antigens. It is associated with poor water metabolism.

Big Picture:

Think of a swamp. Now imagine that the swamp is heated to 98.6 degrees Fahrenheit. This is the human body with water retention. Just as a hot swamp may have swamp gas, mosquitoes, and plenty of fungi, the human body will likewise begin develop poisonous gasses, pathogenic organisms and plenty of fungi.

This is a waterlogged body. Just imagine a city trying to function under two feet of water. Life would go on, but at a very slow pace. This impedes healing and leads to systemic fungal infections.

When this mechanism is predominant, people experience pain that feels heavy; the skin and muscles feel soggy due to water retention, and it is often accompanied with a mental fog. In severe cases it can result in edema.

The treatment strategy for this type of fibromyalgia is to drain the swamp and improve gut balance.

Key Signs:

- Irritable bowel disorder
- Loose stools
- Edema
- Water retention
- Fibro fog
- Symptoms worse in moist or hot weather
- Generalized headache
- Need to remind yourself to drink
- Fatigue
- Chronic fungal infections
- Allergies or chronic sinusitis

Treatment Strategy:

Increase bowel movements and restore healthy gut flora.

We use plant-based interventions to regulate water

metabolism, blood sugar, and blood lipids. It also has immune regulatory effects. We reduce fungi and increase SOD and other antioxidants to help reduce damage caused by inflammation. To combat fibro fog we use herbs that have been shown to increase memory and brain cell proliferation. Because of the influence of gut microbiota on sleep we use the gut flora to help increase 5-HT. The formulas in this category tend to be antibacterial and antiviral and help with pancreatic juice, insulin, and bile secretion.

TYPE THREE: NITRIC OXIDE DYSREGULATION ASSOCIATED WITH ELEVATED CORTISOL

Buildup of nitric oxide associated with sleep deprivation, stress and emotional trauma is associated with chronic pain, stress disorders, and chronic fatigue syndrome.

Big Picture:

Think of a traffic jam. In some areas, you have too many cars; in other areas, there aren't enough. Now replace the cars with a gas that can either help restore homeostasis to the body or cause nerves to disintegrate and you begin to understand the importance of it being distributed safely.

This tends to manifest in two ways based on the fight or flight mechanism.

1. Pain in the shoulders. Fight response. You aren't allowed to punch or claw, which is your natural response; so as it's built up and not used, it creates long-term tension that begins in the shoulders.

2. Pain in the lower back. This is the flight response. Energy surges to the legs, but you have nowhere to run. The tension builds in the lower back.

With the increased oxidation, the liver loses efficiency in catabolizing cortisol, so these stress hormones will build up in the blood stream causing a repeat of traumatic feelings. Initially they have trouble getting to sleep, but as the oxidative damage begins to destroy the liver, kidneys, and nervous system, they will begin waking up around

1:00-3:00 AM and an increase in vivid dreams and in severe cases, nightmares. In an effort to release some of the built-up nitric oxide, the body will tend to cause people to sigh in order to self regulate. With high stress and deregulated nitric oxide, the body suffers nerve pain. It's common to feel pain behind the eyes from a combination of intraocular pressure and oxidative disintegration of the optic nerve. This type of fibromyalgia is associated with dysregulation of melatonin. Melatonin has direct actions on pain signaling.

Key Signs:

- Accompanied with sleep deprivation and insomnia
- Pain which is improved by moving
- Often associated with irritable bowel disorder
- Pain which is worse with sitting and with stress and poor sleep
- Most common cause of fibromyalgia

Treatment Strategy:

Reduce stress, improve sleep, reduce nitric oxide, sigh,

and move lightly to work the tension out of the body. It is also important to address long-term liver damage.

We use plant-based interventions to regulate nitric oxide, reduce stress, regulate melatonin, and improve sleep. We also address liver cirrhosis and regulate gut inflammation to reduce irritable bowel disorder. These interventions have been shown to have a regulatory effect on hormones.

TYPE FOUR: PROSTAGLANDIN DYSREGULATION AND PLATELET ADHESION ASSOCIATED CHRONIC INFLAMMATION AND PAIN

Big Picture:

Think of having a bruise that won't go away. Remember the tenderness and way it fatigued the local muscles. Now extend this bruise to the entire body and mix it with the pain of menstrual cramps or fibroids and you begin to get an idea for how devastating this type of pain can be.

Key Signs:

- Worse in the morning
- Accompanied with morning stiffness
- Sharp, stabbing and wakes people at night
- Improves with increased blood circulation
- Associated with chronic injuries, menstrual disorders, fibroids, and spider veins

Treatment Strategy:

Improve circulation and regulate prostaglandins.

For this type we use sophisticated blends of botanicals that have the following effects:

- Reduce the synthesis of prostaglandins PGs, esp. $PGF_{2\alpha}$ by inhibiting cyclooxygenase 1 (COX). Prostaglandins (PGs) are not only important active mediators in inflammation, but they can also increase the sensitivity of pain. Cyclooxygenase can cause inflammatory mediators such as PGs to release in a large amount.

- Better than morphine for long term pain when compared to morphine they found that short. Some of its pain alleviation may be due to inhibition of the P2X3 receptor.
- Inhibit monoamine oxidase B (MAOB)
- Regulate dopamine.
- Have both glucocorticoid and NSAID inflammatory properties; reduce interleukin 1 beta, 6 and 8 by fibroblasts.
- The sedative effect is as strong as that of 200mg/kg aspirin or 1mg/kg indomethacin
- Wound healing
- Blood vessel formation
- Increase vascular endothelial growth factor (VEGF)
- Increase cellular immunity and significantly reduce markedly elevated interleukin (IL rosette rate).
- Anti-rheumatic capability which is caused by its mediation of lymphocyte proliferation, COX abnormal cell by inhibiting the activation of T helper 1 (Th1) and Th2 cells.

TYPE FIVE: MITCHOCHONDRIAL MYOPATHY

This type of chronic pain is associated with fatigue, low levels of nitric oxide, and muscle weakness. The pain gets worse after movements and is worsened with fatigue. It is often accompanied by immunodeficiency and shortness of breath.

Big Picture:

Being so tired that it literally hurts. The body is too weak to repair itself and regulate pain signals. This pain is typically associated with:

- Fatigue
- Muscle weakness
- Poor wound healing
- The pain gets worse after movements and is worsened with fatigue.
- Often accompanied by immunodeficiency
- Shortness of breath

Key Signs:

- Burning
- Swelling

- Throbbing
- Cramping
- Aching
- Heaviness
- Restless legs
- Leg fatigue

Treatment Strategy:

Boost and regulate nitric oxide, regulate macrophage activity, increase lung capacity, and boost mitochondria.

We use plant-based formulas that have the following effects:

- Increase mitochondria production
- Increase nitric oxide
- Antiviral
- Improve digestive function
- Boost and regulate cellular and humoral immunity
- Anti itching

TYPE SIX: VENOUS INSUFFICIENCY

Big Picture:

Think of being drained of blood. Being pale or cold. Imagine a dying animal having spasms as it bleeds out. Venous insufficiency can cause muscle twitching.

Key Signs:

- Itching and tingling
- Pale complexion
- Fatigue
- Muscle spasms, twitching or restless leg syndrome

Treatment Strategy:

Increase blood production and circulation.

We use plant-based formulas that have the following effects:

- Anti itching
- Anti pain
- Anti tumor
- Anti cancer effects

- Help lower back pain
- Prevent osteoporosis
- Increase red blood cells
- Modulate immune factors
- Increase insulin availability

TYPE SEVEN: DUE TO LOW DHEA'S OR HPA-THYROID DYSREGULATION

This type of fibromyalgia is often associated with thyroid disorders, long-term adrenal response and poor sleep.

Big Picture:

This pain is similar to that of people who go through chemotherapy. Take that and combine it with a loss of sex hormones, then add sleep deprivation and temperature fluctuations.

Key Signs:

- Often seen when fibromyalgia occurs at menopause.
- Associated with estrogen deficiency.
- Associated with night sweats and pain that seems to come from inside the bones.
- Waking in the middle of the night.
- Lumbar pain
- Pain that is worse when standing for long periods
- Poor memory
- Hair loss
- Night sweats

Treatment Strategy:

Sleep well. Enjoy good sleep hygiene by avoiding artificial light at night.

TYPE EIGHT: DYSREGULATION OF ACTH AND CORTISOL ASSOCIATED WITH LUMBAR PAIN AND LOW BODY TEMPERATURE

It usually associated with low libido or sexual dysfunction, nighttime urination, long-term depression and the fear response.

Big Picture:

Think of feeling old and cold. Imagine everything hurting and being afraid of cold weather. Imagine it hurting to stand up and having general aches and pains associated with aging. Now magnify them and bring them on at any age. This creates an understandable cycle of pain and depression.

Key Signs:

- Associated with lumbar pain, and low body temperature
- Associated with low libido or sexual dysfunction, night time urination,
- Often associated with long term depression
- More common in men around andropause

Treatment Strategy:

Warm the body and regulate ACTH and cortisol. Keep a heating pad on the lower back. Strengthen the legs.

Go to Fibrobible.com or Fibrocircle.com and take a quiz to help determine which fibro type is most predominant.

In daily life, we can help adjust all of these through the following ways:

1. Harmonize gut microbiota with the changes in the external environment.

2. Harmonize breathing, thought patterns with the changes in your life.

3. Harmonize relaxation and tensegrity so that every movement serves to massage you and sooth your pain.

Typically pain free within three months and the underlying root is taken care of in nine. Those who seriously devote themselves to treatment may have the pain significantly reduced within a month.

There are three stages to the treatment process:

1. Stop the nerve damage by addressing the root cause.

2. Repair injured nerves.

3. Strengthen the body to prevent future flare-ups.

Alleviating fibromyalgia symptoms in the long run is not only possible, it has been successfully documented for millennia and tested scientifically for the past 50 years. Use of herbal compounds to alleviate the symptoms of fibromyalgia was documented in 280 AD. Since that time, the understanding of fibromyalgia symptoms has developed.

After looking very carefully at different perspectives on healing within the West and East Asia, we discovered some differences in perspective that is endemic to the culture of fibromyalgia in the anglosphere. In order to truly remove this disorder, it is essential to follow these "Ten Commandments of Fibromyalgia". These guidelines may help you to overcome common challenge to transcend the cause of your pain and succeed enjoy a life without flare ups or fibro fog.

THE TEN COMMANDMENTS OF
FIBROMYALGIA

1. No self-pity. All of the energy of anger, fear
   and sadness will now be redirected into
   positive self-care. Whether it's from past
   pain or future fear, it's now over. Your
   focus is now what you can do in this
   moment to feel better and recover.

2. Sleep at night. If sleeping may not be easy,
   then meditate in the dark all night. Artificial
   light derailing your circadian rhythms locks
   you in a pain cycle. Be in the Sun by day
   and in darkness at night. No exceptions.

3. Avoid rapid temperature changes. Dress
   warmer than others. Keep your feet warm
   with slippers when inside. Absolutely no
   iced food or cold drinks. Everything
   ingested will be warm until your pain is
   gone and body is strengthened. Make sure

your hair is dry when leaving the house. Wet hair can cause rapid cooling to the back of the neck and interfere with your lymphatic flow.

4. Reinvest new energy into self-care. Exercising to extremes often leads to relapse. Keep the well primed. It's common for people to become pain free and energetic, and then clean the house and exercise too much. Take a balanced approach and leave yourself with energy for strengthening the internal organs.

5. Cultivate your thoughts. Avoid drama, negativity, media, or music, which is negative or stimulating. Simplify your thoughts and bring the focus of your energy into your body for healing. Let the ripples in your mind pond settle into clarity. As you do this, you can see through the fear of feeling doomed or cursed, and instead, take a rational and step-by-step course toward recovery.

6. Cultivate your gut garden. Use every bite as a choice to heal yourself.

7. Cultivate your breathing. Use it to reduce pain and increase healing.

8. Cultivate your movement. Learn to move with natural poise, posture and grace to make every movement into a massage.

9. Cultivate healthy community. We are social animals and cannot be healthy alone. Create healthy social connections by giving to people who have a positive outlook on life.

10. Pay it forward. The information in this book came to you because for the last few millennia a long chain of people chose to pass it down so you can have relief. As you use these methods to become pain free and energized, share what you have discovered, make it your own, and improve on it for the next generation.

Part I

Chapter 1: An Ancient Legacy

"What has been will be again, what has been done will be done again; there is nothing new under the Sun."

—*Ecclesiastes 1:9*

We once lived by nature's laws. Heaven and Earth were the great makers and destroyers. By the cycles of the sea, we harvested shellfish and set sail. By the seasonal flooding of rivers, we established civilizations. We mastered these rhythms in every step, every breath, every birth, and every death. This is how our ancestors traveled the world, overcame pain, and prevented illness. It is how they strengthened themselves in their journey through life. They passed down this knowledge as a gift to us. It came from one voice to next, carrying new experiences with each generation as it echoed through the ages.

We carry traces of this knowledge today. When we go camping, we learn to avoid berries based on their color and flavor. Rather than memorizing every plant and species, we learn general principles of woodcraft. When we learn to avoid white and bitter berries we are not talking about absolute facts, but rather general tendencies in nature. When we describe spicy food as "hot", we aren't describing its vitamin content. Instead we are describing the way it makes us feel. These experiences formed the foundations of plant-based medicine. Our ancestors discovered that plants could influence human physiology. They could increase water in the body or expel it. They could make people feel warm or clear away inflammation, relieve pain, and help them cool down. They discovered that plants could be used to influence every aspect of human physiology.

At a fundamental level, health is about affecting temperature and moisture in the human body. This seems fairly simple, but it is temperature and moisture that differentiate the Arctic from the Amazon. These temperature variations also have a remarkable effect on which kinds of life these biomes support. A rainforest won't support cacti, scarabs and sidewinder snakes. A desert has very little tolerance for poison dart frogs and banana trees. The lichen of the tundra won't grow in abundance in Ghana. It is the same in the human body. If there is a proliferation of microbiota inside you that isn't to your liking, simply alter your internal temperature and moisture settings to keep them in check.

Looking at the big picture simplifies an overwhelmingly complex challenge. It is impossible to micromanage the trillions of microorganisms within your body or to memorize every chemical structure in a plant, but thankfully, you don't need to. As you discover how to adapt your temperature and moisture, you can change the internal landscape without having to micromanage anything. You can use the flavors, textures and colors to get an overall idea of how plants will affect your body. At an instinctive level you have been doing this all along.

It is the way you choose to warm up with a hearty stew on a cold autumn day or cool off in summer with fresh-cut watermelon. It's as intuitive as taking off your jacket when it's hot. This is the understanding you will be tapping into and exploring. As you read further, there will be a familiarity to all of this. This process is about unlocking instincts you already have and relating them with your own experiences.

The knowledge you will gain from this process will help you to recover faster from illness and maintain optimum fitness. It will allow you to make mistakes and still maintain a fluid balance. You will learn to eat, breathe, and move to adapt to any change. At the beginning stages you can use this knowledge to increase your fitness and mental clarity. With long-term cultivation, you can develop extraordinary abilities.

Today there are practitioners of Tummo meditation who meditate in the freezing Himalayas wearing wet rags to cool themselves down. Wim Hof, a Dutch master, has popularized these skills outside of Asia. He can submerge himself in ice water longer than anyone else on record while maintaining a constant core temperature. He uses this skill to turn harsh landscapes into his playground. He ran a half marathon above the Arctic Circle, barefoot and in shorts. He has ascended mountains like Kilimanjaro and Everest in shorts. He has also demonstrated that he can overcome heat by running a full marathon in the Namib Desert without water consumption. In total he holds 18 Guinness World Records[2]. Over the millennia there have been many accounts in India, China, and Tibet

---

[2] *For further reading on Wim Hof and Tummo meditation, read Becoming the Ice Man | Pushing Past Perceived Limits by Wim Hof and Justin Rosales*

of people demonstrating similar abilities. These people aren't supernatural. They are simply inheritors of ancient survival systems. This knowledge is already within you, waiting to be unlocked.

This book is simply about regaining the abilities already hardwired into your instincts. They are inscribed into your nervous system. By connecting to your instincts you can improve your fitness, resistance to disease, and mental clarity. In reality, these so-called secrets are well known to your average badger. They are the basic skills required for living on Earth. It is how a squirrel runs in parabolic waves. It is the way horses and bears heal themselves with plants after tasting them. It is how wild animals stay adjusted to extreme temperatures. You are already aware of these abilities, you just haven't thought about them at a conscious level.

You already know how you breathe when you suddenly hit cold water. The instinctive gasp into your chest is how your body responds to the sudden shock of cold water. You know this from your experience and inside of that experience, there is a key to understanding how to use breathing to warm the body and begin transforming fat into heat and usable energy. With a little guidance, you can regain these forgotten instincts and use them to become pain free and grow stronger by the day.

As strength fills your muscles, you will naturally feel like moving. This is a great time to begin exploring the forces that are constantly moving through you. When you take a step, waves of force spiral through your body. They undulate and curve through you. When these waves stop at points of internal tension, they cause forces to abruptly slam into the surrounding tissues. Over time this causes injury. You will discover how to use these forces to massage your body with every step. Using these waves, you can develop greater poise, flexibility, and strength.

You are going to discover how to use eating, breathing and moving to adapt your body and thrive. This will help you to develop the kind of fluid strength and instinctive healing found in wild animals. This process is about rediscovering forgotten instincts and tapping into ancient knowledge bases.

It starts with a simple understanding already infused into cultures throughout the world. You are made of

Heaven and Earth – a delicate combination of gases and microbial dust merged into an elegantly integrated whole.

Chapter 2: The Garden of Microbiota

"Then the LORD God formed a man from the dust of the ground..."

—*Genesis 2:7*

You are a part of a great expanse of life. It travels from rolling fields to your most hidden veins. Trillions of fungi, protozoa, and bacteria form a living dust. They form the foundation for Earth's ecosystems. They swim in the dark depths of the sea and reach up into the stratosphere. They permeate every aspect of your existence.

From the time you were born, through all the seasons of your life, they have been with you. They have sustained you and protected you. They have helped you digest food and fight diseases. They have influenced your thoughts and your gut feelings.

Your digestive tract is lined with 100 million neurons. This enteric nervous system shares many of the same neurotransmitters as your brain. The connection they form is called the gut-brain axis. It's how your gut and brain communicate.

Your enteric nervous system interacts directly with microbiota, but also with your emotions. Your emotions affect your hormones. Your hormones directly influence your digestion. Feeling good can make you digest better. If you are digesting well it can also make you happier because healthy digestion sends signals to your brain to make you feel good.

When your gut and brain are working together you can trust your gut cravings to provide you with everything you need. Your trillions of microbial friends see to the details and you respond emotionally. This is a symbiotic relationship that helps you work as an integrated whole. It's only when you lose this harmony that your cravings start to get weird. In some cases they can contribute to some very illogical behavior.

If your gut loses balance, microbiota become parasitic; they can contribute to intestinal lesions, anxiety, stress, food addiction, and a growing list of mental illnesses. This is particularly troubling because microbiota can be quite active in taking control of their environment. They do their best to thrive and spread their cultures as far as possible. If the growing conditions aren't right, they can influence your body to better suit themselves. Microbiota can colonize you just as people have colonized the planet. The earth's landscape bears witness to millennia of human interaction. This ability to alter the environment allowed human populations to spread and flourish.

Microbiota are trying to do the same thing inside of you right now. Some of them have evolved to farm your body by changing your internal climate. They begin to develop your internal garden of microbiota into a landscape better suited for themselves. They are so good at it, they don't need to toil in fields or dig ditches – they can simply program you to feed them what they want. It's as if they are ordering take-out and having it delivered right to their door.

They can manipulate your opioid receptors to make you crave the foods they like. They don't care that it hurts you at a systemic level. When you eat what these microbiota want, they train you by making you depressed. Later, when you eat what they want, they give you a reward of the same opioids that contribute to feelings of social attachment, happiness, and love. It's the same mechanism behind drug addiction. As much as we'd like to imagine that we are too smart for them, it really doesn't matter. Emotion, rather than logic, is the true motivating force behind feeding behavior. This can affect your pain response and even your personality.

Cats carry a parasite called toxoplasmosis. It's a good thing for cats to have. When it spreads to other animals it makes hunting them easy. It hijacks dopamine and makes the prey attracted to cat urine. As long as the cat urinates it is sending out signals that are attracting its food supply. It's a very elegant system, but the trouble is that humans can catch it as well. Researchers estimate that 20–80 percent of humans may have the toxoplasmosis parasite, depending on their exposure to cats. It increases dopamine, which makes people really happy to be around cats. Our love of cats may be in part a programmed response. We might like cats not only because they are cute, but maybe because we are their food. With the exception of domestic house cats, big cats like leopards and tigers tend to consider primates such as humans, monkeys, and chimpanzees to be food. It benefits cats to make us love them. It suckers us into a proximity where they can eat us.

Toxoplasmosis goes a little further. It helps the predator by making its prey less physically coordinated and mentally acute. The parasite does this by jacking up dopamine levels. This makes people feel cuddly and cozy, but having too much can be a problem. It is associated with a lowered attention span and schizophrenia. Toxoplasmosis has also been linked with car accidents and nonfatal suicide attempts in women.

Keep in mind that we are talking about the influence of only one microorganism. It doesn't even qualify as the tip of the iceberg when it comes to the relationship between microbiota and human behavior. For every human living on the planet, there is an estimated 10 million trillion microbes. Some of them have yet to make contact with human beings. What they will bring is anyone's guess.

How they will influence you depends on your internal biodiversity. With a healthy microbiome their influence will be negligible. If you sow wheat in an empty field, you can expect to reap a crop in a few months. If you go into the forest and begin scattering wheat seed, you aren't going to produce a field of grain. Most of those seeds will rot, either in the forest or in the gut of an animal. The few that sprout will have very tough competition. The same is true for pathogenic species in your gut. Biodiversity is your best defense.

BIODIVERSITY

Every garden has its share of bugs[3]. You can either poison them to oblivion or try to maintain a system of checks and balances. There is a time and place for both approaches. In the long run, biodiversity is one of the best forms of pest control. A study at Washington State University found that creating more insect competition served two purposes. The first was that it kept the insects from eating too much; they couldn't treat the garden like a salad bar when they had to watch their little insect backs. The second was that their bug battles resulted in fresh fertilizer for the plants. The plants with insects grew better than controls which used conventional pesticides. Instead of being eaten by the insects, the plants ended up benefiting from them. This can teach us a great deal about gardening the gut and how you look at "bad" microbes.

[3] *Not all insects are bugs. I used this term because it's used for some insects and colloquially for microbial disease.*

Given the right context, they can be beneficial.

INTERNAL ECOLOGY

Wolves are scary. A small wolf can overcome and devour a very strong man. A pack of them in a city park could take out a suburban family with the kind of leisure you might enjoy at a picnic. If they were loose, you would definitely change the frequency of your park visits. You would also think of them as vile enemies if you saw them eating your offspring. Elk share the same sentiments. When wolves are around, elk hide in the brush under the dark forest canopy. If you take wolves out of the picture, it can have dramatic effects on the whole environment.

Yellowstone Park was established in 1872 as a nature preserve. At the same time the government had pressure from farmers who were suffering great losses as wolf populations grew fat on their livestock. Imagine if wolves made daily withdrawals from your bank account, stole your car, and then ate your dog. You would probably want them gone. These government-sponsored extermination policies offered cash for wolf pelts. This program offered ranchers supplemental income and helped them recoup their losses. After a few decades the wolves were gone. Over the next 70 years the effects of a missing species had a dramatic impact on the park.

With the wolves gone, the elk were free to go where they wanted. They relaxed and ventured into the open. For the elk, the American dream was alive and well. They started their own baby boom. They spent family outings by the river munching on tree saplings. One outcome: increased erosion. The rivers became less winding, decreasing surface area and reducing the microclimates and aquatic sanctuaries necessary to sustain life. The park's biodiversity was on a crash course.

To help take over where the wolves left off, people began hunting the elk. This helped to some degree. Despite their best efforts, however, the hunters made terrible wolves. They neglected many wolf duties. For one, they weren't scary enough. They killed the elk, but did so humanely. This didn't stress the elk out enough to alter their digestion or grazing behavior. The elk continued to eat tree saplings without fear and continued to erode the riverbanks.

From the 1970s to the 1990s, public perception of wolves began to change. Films like *Dances with Wolves* began to inspire conservation efforts. Yellowstone National Park and Central Idaho initiated an environmental impact statement designed to reintroduce wolves into the park.

In 1995, park rangers released the wolves. With bands of roaming death lurking just out of scent, the elk were too busy hiding to mate and their birthrate plummeted. Coyotes were also in for a surprise. After the wolves arrived, their population fell by 50 percent. With many coyotes dead, hares and rodents started to prosper. Birds of prey responded to the inviting environment and hung in the sky waiting for their chance to strike. In response, the rodents began burrowing into the earth. Their holes aerated the soil, changing the conditions for microbes, seeds, and plants throughout the ecosystem.

Beaver colonies expanded from one in 2001 to nine in 2011. Beavers are quite industrious with their water conservation projects, and the extra water created wetlands and ponds. Water plants grew. Fish swam among them. Water skippers glided over the glassy water. Otters and birds joined the party to splash around and enjoy some snacks. Moose munched on the water plants. By simply being themselves, wolves helped restore the ecosystem.

When it comes to your internal ecology, bacteria are no more evil than wolves or elk. Every creature has its nature, from those that run and hide to those that aggressively kill. An ecosystem requires both to maintain balance. Some of the most destructive forces are also the greatest sustainers of life.

Chapter 3: Learning from Fungi

"Fungi are the grand recyclers of the planet and the vanguard species in habitat restoration."

—*Paul Stamets*

Fungi are critical to plant life and the overall health of a forest. They break down dead matter and help life to spring anew. They are at once some of largest organisms on the planet and the smallest.

Fungi are diverse and can eat a wide range of toxic materials. Some can eat heavy metals, plastic, and toxic waste. After the tragic nuclear fallout in Chernobyl, radiotrophic fungi began to restore the environment. They used their pigment melanin to convert radiation into chemical energy.

Fungi are capable of restoring order in ways we are just beginning to understand. They are among the more chemically active substances on our planet. The right fungi can serve as medicines, while having the wrong ones can make you hallucinate or even prove to be fatal. They are powerful and prolific. Their spores are everywhere – yes, even in your body.

You can't control the spores in the air, but you can influence the growing conditions within your body. The types of fungi you grow will depend on the overall growing conditions in your gut. To understand how to cultivate fungi inside of yourself, it's good to go foraging for mushrooms. If you have the opportunity, it is not only a great way to get fresh air, food and exercise; it can teach you an incredible amount about the living context of decay and renewal.

My sister Ann is brilliant at hunting and foraging. If she wants mushrooms, she can head straight for them. It's as if there are huge red arrows pointing right at them. By contrast, I wander aimlessly only to find a "mushroom" which inevitably turns out to be a dry leaf. When we go looking for them, I come up short. By the time I manage to find a mushroom, she has bags full. She still considers it a team effort, which is very gracious of her. Of course, I still feel absolutely useless.

I asked her what her secret was. She said something

about luck to make me feel better. It didn't. I knew she was trying to be nice, but I felt that my problem was one of perspective. I asked her about it. She looked at me, perplexed that I could be so oblivious to the world around me. Then she explained it slowly so I could understand. My problem was that I went looking for the mushroom, while she was looking for where the conditions were right for the mushrooms to exist. Fungi spores are everywhere, but they can only grow where the conditions are right. Where pine needles fall, the soil becomes acidic. This becomes an ideal microclimate for the king bolete mushroom. Oak trees provide an altogether different environment that is nourishing to truffles, maitakes and chanterelles. Ann was looking at the context of the forest, while I was looking for a dot in a panorama of camouflage.

As we went on later mushroom expeditions I began to notice that every kind of rotting plant seemed to host its own variety of fungi. If you pile up dead blackberry bushes, they have little mushrooms on them that don't seem to grow on other plants. As I saw the different plants, each with their own kinds of fungi, it reminded me of an article I saw in a medical journal. It concluded that the wider the variety of vegetables we consume, the more diverse the microbiome. It was one thing to read on paper, but it was another to experience in real life. As I ducked under low boughs and avoided thorns, I found myself not only exploring the forest, but also understanding the human body at a deeper level.

Chapter 4: Climates Barriers

"In some sense man is a microcosm of the universe: therefore what man is, is a clue to the universe. We are enfolded in the universe."

—*David Bohm*

CLIMATE BARRIERS

Every creature is confined to its climate. This is why you are unlikely to discover lions in Antarctica or killer whales roaming the African savannah. The same is true for smaller forms of life. When microbiota travel to an inhospitable region, they die. These climates act as barriers that prevent unwelcome microbiota from taking root and thriving. Your body creates a climate barrier by maintaining different ratios of heat and moisture. As long as your body remains distinct from the outside environment, you stay healthy. It's similar to the way you maintain a home.

In a house, you adjust the heat to maintain a microclimate. If a house is well maintained it can last generations, but when no one is around to maintain the home, it can rot within a decade. Windows freeze and thaw. Boards flex and warp as they respond to external changes. Weathered windows shatter as birds smash into them. As the windows fall, the house inhales the outside atmosphere. In moist climates, molds come in with the wet wind and begin rotting the house. Fluctuations in cold and heat further stretch and splinter the wood. These changes in temperature and moisture bring different varieties of microbiota that devour the house in different ways. They quickly turn the house into a hovel. Over the years, it deteriorates from a hovel into an indistinguishable part of the landscape. If you neglect to maintain a climate barrier, you don't go for very long without rotting. If you maintain a distinct barrier, your internal climate can help prevent the microbiota in your environment from breaking you down.

If you are in a damp environment and your feet have water retention, the local microbiota can waltz right in and begin eating them. If your body is hospitable to diseases carried on the crisp autumn winds, you may in fact catch a "cold" from the influenza virus riding those winds into your lungs. If instead your internal microbiome is opposite in nature to the outside environment, then you create a climate barrier.

When properly cultivated, a climate barrier helps you adjust to the outside environment. It makes you comfortable outdoors. You can confidently overcome whatever challenges come your way.

Traditional diets are often designed to help maintain this barrier. Dietary traditions change based on climate. A warmer climate may signal people to eat less, and enjoy a diet of fruits and vegetables. By contrast, a cold environment will signal people to put on fat and cause them to crave rich, hearty foods that warm the body.

In a study on microbiota in children from Africa and Europe, researchers found that African children had bacteria such as *Prevotella* and *Xylanibacter*, which encode genes for breaking down plant sugars. This made sense considering that their diet was rich in fiber, starch, and plant sugars. The European children, by contrast, didn't have these species of bacteria and had diets higher in sugar, starch, and fat, but comparably low fiber. The ratio of bacteria the European children demonstrated is associated with obesity. The European children were eating stodgier foods that tend to warm the body. In contrast, the African children had a higher-fiber plant-based diet. This diet had significantly higher levels of anti-inflammatory molecules. All of these factors caused the African diet to have a more cooling effect on the body, while the European diet was more fattening. These findings make perfect sense when we consider climate. The dietary cultures of Africa and Europe are based on the challenges of their respective environments. In cooler areas of Europe, it makes sense to be insulated. In warmer climates, where additional insulation and heat can contribute to heat stroke and other illnesses, this same level of fat can be very harmful.

THE EFFECTS OF CLIMATE ON THE HUMAN BODY

Just as trees sigh in the wind and seaweed undulates in the ocean, you too are subject to natural rhythms. Your body changes with the climate and weather. Changes in temperature and moisture affect blood circulation and hormone production. The conditions in the outside environment will influence what you come into contact with. This can greatly influence your health, memory, and even your personality. The weather affects everyone. By studying how it affects you, you can better understand how to adapt to change.

HEAT

There are three main sources of heat in the human body:

-Heat produced from the metabolism of human cells

-Heat produced from the metabolisms of microbiota

-Heat you absorb from radiation.

Warm soup, sunshine, and a crackling fire can all introduce heat into the body. They work in concert to heat you from within. When you feel too hot, you lose your appetite. This is because the process of digestion generates heat. Your body doesn't want you to overheat so it reduces your appetite to help you cool down. To further avoid overheating, it makes you feel tired to keep you from moving too much. The heart begins pumping hard to send blood circulation to the surface of the body where it can cool off. This can contribute to heat rash and makes heat particularly dangerous for those with heart problems. Because your body wants to reduce its metabolism and get water, you naturally feel more inclined to eat fruits and vegetables to stay hydrated and cool off. These foods require your body to do less work compared to eating peppery beef jerky. Your body cools down when you breathe, sweat, urinate, and defecate. The faster these processes happen, the easier it is to cool down.

COLD

When you feel cold, your body does its best to avoid heat loss. Your body reduces circulation to the extremities. By closing down external circulation, it increases your blood pressure. It's the same as putting your thumb over the nozzle of a hose to make it spray farther. To avoid raising blood pressure, your body reduces the blood volume by making you pee more and reducing thirst. Instead of feeling thirsty, your body will signal you to eat more. In this way, the process of digestion can help warm you up. When the weather is cold, fruits and vegetables become less appealing compared to heavier foods. It would seem logical that cold exposure would inspire you to start exercising, but this isn't always the case. Cold exposure often signals your body to feel lazy so it can store fat to insulate you for long-term survival.

DAMP

When it is hot, you sweat to cool yourself down. As the water dries, it wicks away heat. Unfortunately when the weather is humid, the sweat takes a long time to dry so you don't cool down as easily. When it is cold, humidity makes you cold and wet. It wicks heat away from your body. It makes you feel as if the damp is soaking into your body. Life follows water. When the air is humid, microbes ride the airborne water droplets. Some of them are friendly, but others just want to eat you. Your immune system has to fight them off. All of this self-defense can take its toll. This is part of the reason why humid weather can make people feel foggy, tired, and lethargic. When it comes to regulating the microbiome, controlling water metabolism is the most important thing. Think of your house. If you have a flooded room, it doesn't matter if you turn on the heater. Without actively removing the water, the house will get moldy and rot. The same is true of the human body. When water is where it shouldn't be, it causes overgrowths of microbiota that become pathogenic.

DRY

As people age, they dry out. When people are born, they are moist and warm; when they are close to death, they are often dry and cold. This is part of the natural life cycle.

To alleviate many symptoms of aging and prolong life, it can be helpful to study the effects of oxidation and inflammation. Oxidation means rusting, and inflammation means fire, and it is through these two forces that things tend to get destroyed in dry weather. Whether it's a person, sagebrush, or an old Chevy, dryness uses rust and fire to return everything to dust.

Oxidation and inflammation are associated with aging. There are theories that oxidation is actually the cause of aging [4]. Oxidation is an important part of human physiology. It is a byproduct of healthy metabolism, and certain oxidants are important signaling molecules. You can think of oxidation like heat and anti-oxidation like

[4] *Does imbalance cause inflammation-oxidation or does the inflammation-oxidation promote imbalance? I'm hesitant to agree that it is the single cause of aging, but rather I believe it contributes to maintaining an underlying imbalance.*

cold. I use this metaphor because oxidation occurs with heating inflammation, and plants with the highest antioxidants tend to be bitter, sour and cooling. Research has demonstrated that bitter and sour plants have higher antioxidant levels than pungent and sweet plants. In addition, sour and bitter plants tend to contain anti-inflammatory compounds. In traditional Chinese medicine, these plants are considered cooling. They are not intrinsically good, but if there is heat, dryness, and oxidation-inflammation, they may be helpful.

Neither oxidation nor anti-oxidation is superior. The body requires a balance of both. Oxidative stress is what happens when you get too much heat and not enough metaphorical coolant. This affects the cells in your regulatory systems; your body can't regulate itself, and it's easy to get unbalanced. Oxidative rusting influences the nervous, endocrine, and immune systems. It not only wears these systems down, it prevents them from communicating. That's really bad. No injury is that big of a deal if you can bounce back and maintain your natural balance, but once these regulatory centers are affected, you never can quite heal like you used to. When you start to tip off-balance and can't return to normal, you begin a downward spiral that ends in death. Everyone dies; death is not the real issue here. The real tragedy is not living well. When your regulatory systems can't return to balance, life becomes painful and difficult. People lose memory, hormone balance, even themselves. They forget loved ones, suffer mood swings, and can become difficult to live with. For most people, this is scarier than death. You really don't want your last years on Earth to be stressful and weird for everyone around you.

THE EFFECT OF CLIMATE ON PLANTS

Plants and animals develop attributes that help them adapt to their climates. You can benefit from these adaptations. High-altitude plants develop properties to help themselves respire. If you want an herb to help with breathing and oxygen intake, high-altitude plants are a great place to look. High-altitude plants such as Tibetan Rhodiola increase hemoglobin. This helps you hold more oxygen in your blood and prevents altitude sickness. Not all high-altitude plants have this effect, but understanding how plants adapt to their environment narrows the places you need to look. If you want a plant that can help you warm up, look in a cool climate. If you need to cool down, look for plants that come from warmer climates.

In the hot and wet tropics, you can find herbs with antibacterial and antifungal properties (these types of plants are typically bitter and sour). The entire biome of the tropics is buzzing with microbial life, and the plants that thrive there have adapted by having antibacterial, antifungal, and antioxidant properties to survive. You use many of the same chemical structures as plants. These structures help you adapt to the climate. You can often make use of a plant's lifetime of hard work when you ingest it.

Chapter 5: Cultivate the Garden Within

"Then the Lord God took the man and put him into the Garden of Eden to cultivate it and keep it."

—*Genesis 2:15*

You don't need to pull out a syringe and get a sap sample to see that a tree needs water. You only need to look at withered leaves to see that it is too dry. Your body will also give you signs of its internal condition if you know where to look.

By observing outward signs and combining them with an intuitive feeling for your body you can better understand yourself and take steps to cultivate your internal garden. The first step is to stick out your tongue and see what it has to teach you.

TONGUE: WINDOW TO THE GUT

Look at your tongue to get an overall idea of your digestive health. Pay attention to the color and shape of the tongue body. Consider the thickness, distribution, and color of the tongue's coating. A healthy tongue has a pink tongue body with an even thin, white or clear coating.

Tongue

	Dry Cold	**Dry Hot**	**Damp Hot**	**Damp Cold**
Color of Tongue Body	Pale	Red	Red	Pale
Shape	Fat	Thin	Thin	Fat
Coating	Thin	Thin	Thick	Thick
Color of Tongue Coating	White	Yellow	Yellow	White

Tongue Color

Pale: Sign of cold and possibly anemia

Light red: Sign of health

Bright red: Sign of inflammation

Slightly purple: Sign of lack of oxygen or cardiovascular disease. Associated with strokes and heart attacks.

Shape: As a muscle, the tongue's shape can change. If you stick out your tongue and it is stiff, it becomes triangulated, while it's more of an oval when relaxed. When inspecting the tongue make sure that it is relaxed.

Thin tongues: Sign of longstanding dryness.

Fat tongues: Sign of water retention and/or digestive weakness.

Ridges: Ridges on the sides are caused by the tongue is pressing against the teeth. If there is water retention the tongue will lose its shape and form to the teeth. It's similar to how you can press into the leg of someone with edema and the thumbprint will leave an impression. This indicates water retention.

Short tongues: Typically a sign of deficient fluids.

Long: Typically a sign of heat.

Tongue Coating

No coating: A sign of heat **Light thin or clear coating:** Healthy

Thick coating: Food retention or dampness **Geographic**

tongue: Complex pattern. See a TCM doctor[5].

Cracks (Fissured): Like dry earth, it is a sign of either a lack of fluids or the improper distribution of fluids.

---

[5] *This pattern is caused from complex and specific imbalances between the endocrine system and the gut.*

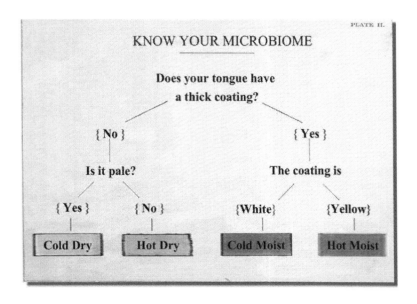

UNDERSTANDING THE FACE

SKIN

Red: Heat

Pale: Cold

Dry: Dry

Oily: Damp

EYES

Bloodshot or red: Heat

Clear and shiny: Healthy

Bags: Poor digestion or immune response

Dark circles: Water retention

LIPS

Red: Heat

Pale: Cold/anemic

Dark/Purple: Poor circulation

STOOLS

Observation of the stool is one of the easiest ways to get an idea about the health of your microbiome. Stools should be formed, easy to pass and medium brown in color. The smell should not be overly strong. Passing stools should be comfortable without any sensations of pain, burning or urgency. It's normal to have slight variations in the stool based on dietary changes.

	Dry Cold	**Dry Hot**	**Damp Hot**	**Damp Cold**
Consistency	Dry	Dry	Loose	Loose
Size	Normal	Smaller	Normal	Normal
Smell	Less Smell	Foul Smell	Foul Smell	Mildly Sweet
Undigested Food	Yes	No	No	Yes
Mucus	None	None	Yellow	Clear or White
Sticky (requiring more tissue)	No	No	Yes	Yes

COLOR:

Brown: Normal.

Green: Too much bile is being released.

Black: Usually nothing; black and tarry can indicate upper GI tract bleeding.

Red blood: Likely a hemorrhoid, but get it checked out by a doctor.

Chapter 6: Understanding Food

"He who distinguishes the true savor of his food can never be a glutton; he who does not cannot be otherwise."

—Henry David Thoreau

SINGLE FLAVORS

The ratio of flavors in a single food can help you determine how that food will affect your levels of heat and moisture.

Plants change based on climate. They adapt based on the soil and climate. One book might say that a grapefruit is sour and another might say it is bitter or sweet, and all of them will be correct, depending on the grapefruit itself.

A single food will come with a combination of flavors. The presenting flavor will be the most predominant. Based on the major flavors you can get an idea of how the food will affect you. This isn't an absolute law, but rather a general principle that works out more often than not.

Everyone will experience taste slightly differently. This

is in part due to differences in microbiota and taste genes. If your ancestors lived in an area where a particular flavor was associated with poison, then being averse to that flavor would have helped them survive. Not every group of people has the same taste preferences. Not everyone digests in the same way. There are general rules, but how you fine-tune this information will ultimately be based on how you experience sight, taste, and texture. This is the easiest way to determine what is chemically available and how it will influence your body.

OVERVIEW

Pungent/Spicy – Warming, associated with killing anything trying to invade the body and increasing immune function

Sweet – Nourishing and moistening, increases body size

Sour – Cool and moist, astringing and holding

Bitter/Bland – Draining, cooling, reduces body size

Salty – Softening, moistening

PUNGENT/SPICY – WARMS AND PROTECTS

Pungent or spicy food tends to be warming. Think of biting into horseradish or wasabi and the feeling of heat lifting into your sinuses. Imagine eating chili peppers until you break a sweat. These foods have a tendency to increase nitric oxide and boost the immune system. Pungent and spicy foods typically contain volatile oils, amino acids, organic acids, glycosides and alkaloids. If you are feeling cold, foods with this flavor can help you adapt. Not all pungent plants are warming, but as a general rule, it works out.

Arugula	Sichuan peppercorn	Patchouli leaves
Chard	Clove	(huo xiang)
		Cilantro
Collards	Chili pepper	
Daikon	Cinnamon	Mustard greens
Ginger	Pepper	
Chives	Dill seed	
Garlic	Star anise	

Pungent foods:

These are the flavors that seem to rise into your head and set fire to your nose. Wasabi, garlic, and horseradish will all clear the sinuses and a high enough dosage can cause sweating. If you have ever seen people eat dangerously spicy food, you can remember the redness of their faces, the tears, and the sweating. If you didn't know better, you would think they had just come from a long journey in the desert.

I distinctly remember the first time I saw a man drink an entire bottle of hot sauce. This wasn't your grocery-store hot sauce; it was the kind you buy at hot sauce competitions. A man came into my friend's restaurant looking for a job. He was a vagrant with a passion for spice. He produced a bottle with a warning label from one of his pockets. It suggested two to three drops and had the words "medical attention" on the disclaimer. In an effort to endear himself to his potential employer, he decided to drink it. All of it. We tried to stop him, but honestly, we didn't try that hard. We were all a bit shocked and morbidly curious. He seemed fine at first, but soon his face was red and his eyes became bloodshot. Within a minute, he was slumped into a corner. We were a little concerned and asked if he needed bread or to go see a doctor. He held up his hand with the palm outward, but it was difficult to discern his meaning. It could have meant, "No, I'm fine" or "For the love of God, please help". It was hard to tell because he was panting as though he was trying to expel heat with every breath. The redness of his face, the dryness of his lips, and the dead, bloodshot eyes seemed like they belonged to a desert-dwelling lizard more than to a man. A half hour later, he came around to the point that he could stand up and speak. He seemed genuinely shocked to discover that he hadn't been hired. He asked to spend the night at my friend's house and was once again denied. He was a man short on many things, but fire wasn't one of them.

Even if you have never eaten a chili pepper in your life, you can get a good idea of what it does by its color and flavor. It's spicy and red. Both of these are good indicators that it will be warming. These general rules of color and flavor taught our ancestors to figure out the basic properties of plants.

To ancient people, anything that increased heat, circulation, metabolism, and heart rate could be considered fire. They recognized little practical difference between peppery foods, a hot day, a warm fire, or hard physical work. The end result was the same. On a cold day, you could move, drink liquor, or stand by the fire to warm up. This was the common sense of humanity before climate control. Over time, people discovered that certain foods warmed the body, while others left them feeling colder.

They maintained internal homeostasis by combining moistening foods with drying foods and matching warming and cooling foods so that they could enjoy both without causing the gut to lose its fundamental balance. When the weather changed, they could adjust this balance to allow for fluctuations in heat and moisture.

SWEET – NOURISHES AND MOISTENS

In nature, sweet means that you have hit the jackpot. These foods are rare in a natural setting. Your body loves sweet foods and will try to get as much nourishment from them as possible. If you have something sweet every day, you should consider yourself in paradise. Sweet foods tend to contain sugar. I know, not a big surprise there, but keep in mind how rare that is in nature. Humans are instinctively drawn toward sweet foods, but too much sweet food can lead to a swampy internal environment. Naturally sweet foods typically contain sugars, saponins, proteins, amino acids, vitamins and sterols. They tend to boost the immune system, provide energy to the body and have a very slight influence on raising body temperature.

Sweet foods:

Asparagus	Orange zest	Carrot
Sugar	Spinach	Honey
Stevia	Pumpkin	Mushroom
Monk fruit	Squash	Huang qi
Astragalus	Sweet potato	Dates
Corn	Plantain	Longan Fruit

SOUR – COOLS, HOLDS AND RETAINS

The word "acidus" in Latin means sour. With a few exceptions, sour foods determine acidity. Sour flavors are often found in vegetables and fruit. They cool the body and increase bile to help break down fats. Sour foods are where you tend to find organic acids, tannins and glycosides which increase gastrointestinal movement, and promote gastric acid, bile and saliva.

Sour foods:

Citrus fruits	Dandelion greens	Chinese hawthorn
Green apples	Sauerkraut	(shan zha)
Vegetables	Tomato	Grapes
		Apricot

BITTER – DRAINS AND COOLS

Bitter foods tend to be poisons. Some of these poisons are designed to kill animals. These plants typically are poisonous to humans. Other bitter plants are designed to kill smaller forms of life. This is why many bitter plants are antifungal, antibacterial and antiviral. These make excellent medicines and are useful for cooling the body down as they slow the metabolism in your microbiome. At low doses they have regulatory actions on the microbiome. They can help clean your intestines and reduce inflammation. Bitter foods usually contain alkaloids and amaroids. They tend to lower blood pressure and blood sugar. Overall they are useful for clearing inflammation, draining water, and clearing the intestines.

Bitter foods:

Bitter melon	Cranberries	Pu-er tea
Romaine heart	Cocoa	Buckwheat
Kale	Ku ding tea	

BLAND – DRAINS AND REDUCES

In nature, bland foods are the rule. If you were foraging for food, the majority of your diet would be bland. Fibrous roots, tubers, and mushrooms tend to have a bland flavor. Today we dislike bland; we spice it up, sweeten it, and otherwise try to make it interesting. Still, a bland diet is the best for overall health.

Bland foods tend to cause urination and lower blood pressure. They also help to maintain even blood sugar. Their fiber creates a time-release function for sugar so that your body can process it efficiently. Most bland foods are also slightly bitter. If you are having trouble finding bland foods, then you can add psyllium husk and other fiber sources to your diet. This is an easy way to increase the fiber-to-sugar ratio, which has a similar effect to increasing bland foods. Some more palatable bland-flavored foods are beta-glucan foods.

Bland foods:

Oats	Rice	Spinach
Barley	Pearl barley	Eggplant
Yeast	Red beans	River fish
Cattails	Winter melon	Green beans
Mushroom and	Cabbage	
Fungi	Bok choy	

BETA GLUCAN FOODS

Beta-glucans are sugars found in the cell walls of graminaceous crops such as barley, rye and oats. They are also found in bacteria, fungi and edible mushrooms. They have displayed anti-diabetic activities and have been shown to lower cholesterol. Coix seed, also known as Job's tears, are a bland and slightly bitter grain used in Asia for drying and cooling the internal gut garden in order to reduce pain caused by gut dysbiosis.

SALTY – RETAINS WATER, SOFTENS HARDNESS, CAUSES DRYNESS

When it comes to plants, the easiest way to determine if one is salty is whether it causes thirst. Watermelon quenches thirst, whereas cherries make you want to drink water. By this we can conclude that watermelon is sour and sweet, and cherries are sour, sweet, and salty. Where salt goes, water follows, so a high salt diet will eventually lead to water retention and high blood pressure. Salty foods usually contain inorganic salts, proteins and amino acids.

Salty foods:

Seafood

Cherries (also sweet and sour) (again, don't take the examples too seriously.)

Black beans

Pork

To push outward and protect

Enjoy pungent, bland and bitter foods that are nutritionally sparse.

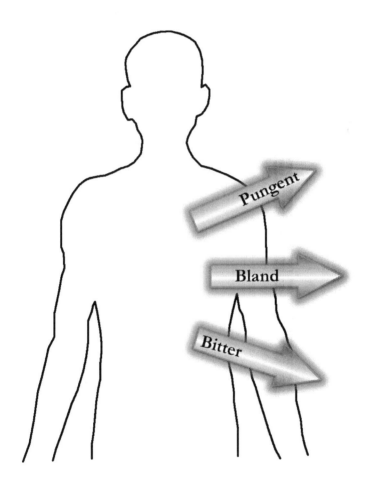

To draw inward and nourish

Enjoy sweet, sour and salty foods that are nutritionally dense.

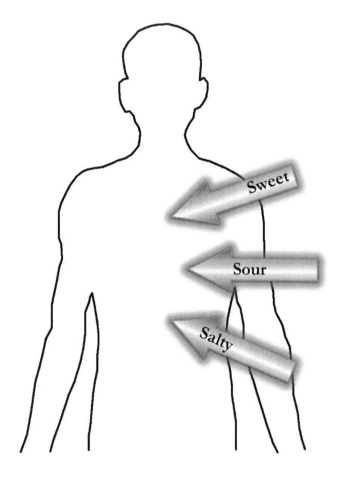

FLAVOR COMBINATIONS

Pungent + Salty = Warming and moistening

Salty+ Sour = Cooling and moistening

Bitter + Pungent = Warming and drying

Bitter + Sour = Cooling and drying

BALANCING MOISTURE

DRY HEAT VS. DAMP HEAT (CHECK THIRST)

You will know that water retention is worse than the heat if there is no desire to drink water. In those cases, first expel water using warming teas known for settling the stomach, for example, pu-er tea.

If heat is worse than the dampness, there will be constant thirst. In these cases, inflammation is the primary concern, so bitter teas such as bitter melon and ku ding tea are more appropriate. Once the thirst is alleviated, see to warming and drying the digestive system with bland and pungent foods.

Forgetting damp heat

During my first summer in Chengdu I found myself unbearably hot. It wasn't the type of heat I was accustomed to. Having spent summers in Mexico and Southern California without air conditioning I thought I had it down. You open the windows at night, tinfoil the windows, create airflow over wet rags. I had all of the tricks that work very well in an arid climate, but they were perfectly useless in Chengdu. Surrounded by mountains, the city has wet moisture hanging over it like a wet wool blanket. The air doesn't flow. It causes a heavy feeling and people cope by sleeping more. After a few weeks I began to get a little heat fatigue. This dropped my IQ by about 60 points. I wasn't thirsty and had to remind myself to drink. With my impaired judgment, I forgot that this was a classic sign of dampness. I had cooling bitter teas. Due to my heatstroke logic, I was rewarded with stomach pain and diarrhea. I took some herbs which warm digestion and caused me to sweat. Once I was able to sweat I felt thirst and gradually regained normal water metabolism and digestive health. For the next few days I ate more ginger in the morning to warm digestion and went for a daily run to break a sweat and improve water metabolism. Within the week I felt mentally clear and enjoyed a feeling of strength that made me want to get out and exercise.

DAMP COLD VS. DRY COLD (CHECK URINE)

You can tell that dampness is worse than cold by the frequency of urination. If dampness is worse, urine will be hesitant and tend to be frothier. If there is dry cold, people tend to experience more frequent urination.

Forgetting Damp Cold

When I was still in Chinese medicine school, my friend Biagio was getting married and he asked me to be the best man. I booked a flight from Vancouver, BC, to South Dakota to meet him. I had a bit of cold when I headed out and found myself hungry and waiting for my connecting flight in Denver. The airport didn't have many healthy options. Food was either fried or raw, and neither one seemed appropriate. My tongue had a white coating. I was in Denver so I figured that it must be due to the cold environment. Tongues don't tend to change that quickly, but I was pretty new at this. I thought that I would warm up my cold with some spicy tortilla soup. When it arrived I found that it had more oil than I had expected, but I thought that the spices would counter it. Unfortunately I was wrong. The problem was that cold wasn't the primary challenge; it was that the damp-loving microbiota of the Pacific Northwest had found their way into my lungs. The oil further moistened my system and allowed them to spread.

It went from being an illness I could have easily overcome with diet to something a little more serious. My throat became sore and it hurt to swallow or speak. This ruined the speech I had planned. I was swollen and in pain. It was a traditional Lakota wedding, beautiful in every detail. Everyone was crying tears of joy, while I was crying tears of pain. I'm pretty sure that many people suspected as much because they joked about it when we watched the wedding video. While everyone was shaking hands and hugging, there was an understandable hesitation when people got to me since I was clearly diseased. I ended up at a local clinic getting a big needle full of antibiotics into my backside. I had considered heat and cold without considering moisture. It was a painful lesson, a funny memory and a mistake I wouldn't make again.

Adjusting Moisture

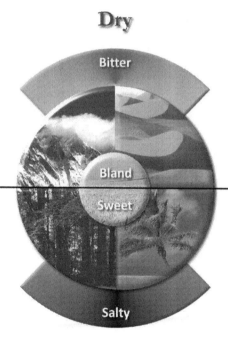

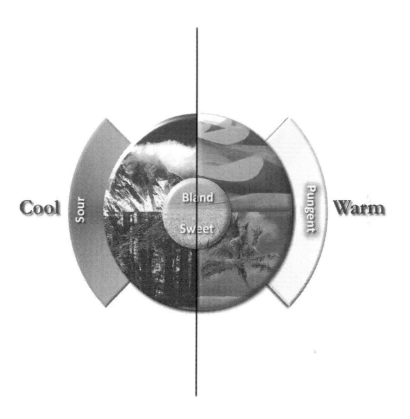

Adjusting Temperature

Cool

Sour

Bland

Sweet

Pungent

Warm

Dry Cold vs. Dry Heat

You either feel hot or cold.

Dry Cold vs. Wet Cold

Your lips and nose get dry with dry cold.

Forgetting Temperature

During my first year of Chinese medicine school I started to learn about how to alter my microbiome using food. I knew I had dampness. I was in a damp environment and my tongue had a thick, white coating. I started eating lots of coix seeds and pearl barley. The book said that it was good for dampness. They had a bitter and bland flavor and did in fact cause me to start draining off extra water. It caused me to urinate a lot, but really didn't help that much. Being inexperienced, I decided that perhaps I wasn't eating enough of it and began having it with every meal. I ended up feeling cold, groggy and lazy as my microbiome continued to get damp. I started to put on fat around the waist. I was making my gut too cold. Without any warming activity in the gut, it had lost its ability to efficiently metabolize water. Without enough heat, my body becomes soggy. After this, I learned that a healthy gut is a slightly warm gut. Once it gets too cold, it becomes like a cold bog that has little hope of ever drying out. I began eating more peppery, spicy and pungent foods to warm the gut. At the time I was intensely focused on studying so my method of cooking was simply to put garlic cloves and a few sweet potatoes in the oven. The combination of pungent and sweet foods caused me to warm up. I began belching more as the balance of gases and microbiota shifted in the gut and I regained balance. I felt strength gradually return to my limbs and pain relief over the next week or so. The cool, damp weather no longer seemed to get into my bones. Instead, it felt comfortable. I began to get out more and exercise. With a healthy climate barrier, I stopped fighting the weather and really begin to feel a part of the landscape.

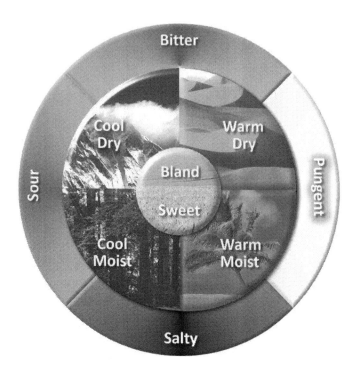

The upper left quadrant is made up of sour and bitter flavors. This will cool and dry the body, making it more like the Arctic. It is ideal to eat foods or herbs that have these flavors if you live in a moist and warm environment or if your internal microbiome has become too tropical.

The upper right quadrant is made up of bitter and pungent flavors. This will warm and dry the body. It will make your internal microbiome more like a desert. This is ideal if you live in a moist and cool region or if your internal microbiome has become too moist and cool.

The lower left quadrant is made up of sour and salty flavors. This will moisten and cool the body, making your body like the Pacific Northwest. This is ideal if you live in a warm and dry climate or if your internal microbiome has become too warm and dry.

The lower right quadrant is made up of pungent and salty flavors. This will warm and moisten the body. It will make your internal microbiome more like the tropics. This is ideal if you live in a cold and dry region or if your internal microbiome has become too cold and dry.

INFLUENCE OF COOKING

The way you prepare a meal will influence its temperature, density, and overall flavor. The properties of a single food aren't that significant because they change once they are cooked. Bananas may be high in potassium, but once they are fried and salted, the effects of them begin to share more in common with pork rinds and potato chips than they do fruit salad. This means that looking at a single ingredient in a single plant tells us nothing about how the food will affect you once the processing is complete. Remember that the strongest flavors will be the most dominant and can give you a good idea of the meal's overall effect; however, the way food is prepared will also change how you digest it. Generally, a lighter density is more drying, and a higher density, such as lard, is more moistening.

Barbecued or dehydrated foods – Relatively warming and drying

Frying – Moistening and warming

Deep fat frying – Relatively warming and moistening

Boiling – Relatively cooling and moistening

Raw – Typically cooling, with the exception of certain wild meats

Foods prepared cold – Generally cooling

MICROCLIMATES IN FOOD TEXTURE

Every substance has its own density and texture. These

textures create microclimates. An increased surface area houses more life, and this changes how fast food can break down. If you toss a log on a compost pile, it will break down slowly. If you first put the log in a wood chipper, it will rot quickly. The way you cut and chew your food will change its rate of decomposition inside your body.

Everything you eat is itself filled with millions of tiny microclimates hosting trillions of microbiota that are actively sharing your food. Even if you cook the food, by the time it cools enough to eat, it is teeming with life. When you eat your food, you enlist the microbiota that are already trying to break it down. It's a joint effort that works out for everyone. The more surface area your food has, the more microclimates there are for microbiota to move in and begin breaking it down. To increase surface area on your food, chop it into smaller pieces and chew thoroughly.

SEASON

Fruit that is ripe in summer defends against the heat so the fruits are more cooling. Animals butchered in winter have more fat and are more warming. In winter, roots and meat are more readily available. In spring, sour shoots and grasses become available. In summer, sweeter fruits ripen. In autumn, apples, squash and grains are in season. Eating seasonally helps you get fresher food which is more suitable for the time, but you don't need to take it too seriously. How that particular plant or animal balanced itself may leave behind chemicals which can help you, but not always. It's just a guideline. The most important thing is the state of your body and how it is interacting with the environment.

PART OF THE ANIMAL

If you want to build a body part, you need the raw materials. If you need to repair something, eating a similar tissue can give you the material you are looking for. If you want stronger bones, have some bone soup. If you have poor intestines, then eat some intestines. It seems primitive, but this idea is used in modern drug therapy.

Several modern medications are derived from animal parts. To have a stronger thyroid, doctors prescribe a medication that originated in a cow's thyroid gland. Using Latin names and modern packaging doesn't change the fact that some pharmaceuticals come from things like horse urine, pig intestines, snake venom, and insects. This doesn't necessarily mean that "eye of newt" will help you see better; these are just general guidelines for nourishing the body.

COLOR

Colors are often useful to help predict a plant's effect. Brighter colors tend to be more warming than those on the darker end of the color spectrum. The warmest color is white, and the coolest is black. Bright red or white berries tend to be the most chemically active and warming, while black, purple and deep blue foods tend to be salty, sour, moist and cooling. Consider flavor first because it is the most reliable indicator. After considering flavor you can observe color to infer what else a food might be good for.

White – White foods are often pungent, and they tend to be more warming. These foods tend to benefit the lungs and immune system. Think of garlic, radishes, and plants that are naturally white.

Red – Red foods are often warming. They tend to affect the blood. They tend to be spicy or bitter and are often poisonous.

Orange – Orange foods tend to be sweet and nourishing.

Yellow – Yellow foods are likewise sweet. Brown foods such as potatoes and brown rice also fall into this category.

Green – Green foods tend to be sour and are generally good for the liver and blood.

Blue – Blue foods are often a combination of sweet and sour. They tend to be good for the liver and blood.

Violet – Purple foods tend to go to the blood. This is true both for poisons and for medicines.

Black – Black foods are often salty or are seeds. These are good for the kidneys and reproductive organs and tend to increase antioxidants. They also tend to be relatively moistening.

THE "WESTERN" DIET

Most foods North Americans enjoy are moistening, and the culinary spices tend to be drying. This isn't a coincidence. These culinary traditions were based on holistic reasoning and plant-based medicine. The modern Western diet is what happens when you forget how to properly season food. The way you combine spices can alter the "season" within. This idea is found in Chinese medicine. Adapting the body using spices is called "turning with the seasons". It allows you to bring summer inside of yourself in the midst of winter or cool yourself in summer. The correct use of seasonings is an easy way to affect your internal climate. As an exercise we can look at many common North American foods and spices using the perspective of how they influence temperature and moisture.

PREDICTING THE NATURE OF FOODS

HAMBURGERS:

If the beef is fried, it will be warming and moistening. If there are pickles, onion and mustard, these will help to dry the moistening properties of the hamburger. If you add mustard, it becomes more warming and drying. Overall the hamburger is warming and moistening. If it's grilled and full of spices and vegetables, it becomes more balanced.

PIZZA:

Generally speaking, thin crust is drying, while thick is more moistening. The toppings will also influence the pizza's properties. Cheese is moistening; peppers are drying. Mushrooms are cooling and drying. There are baked vegetarian pizzas and meat-lover's extra-cheese pizzas that offer many layers of grease. These are among the more dampening and moistening foods available.

SODA:

The cold temperature and sugar overload bears down on digestion. At best, soda is cooling and moistening.

CHICKEN TENDERS:

Warming and moistening.

FRENCH FRIES/TATER TOTS:

They are fried and starchy, so they are warm and moistening. When combined with ketchup or mayonnaise they become overly moistening for most people.

TACOS:

There are two main types of tacos: Mexican and American. Traditional tacos come with plants. If you pick up a taco in a plaza in Mexico, you could expect to find a corn tortilla filled with cilantro, radish, lime and a little bit of meat. This type of taco is pretty balanced. The spicy sauce with it would help to warm digestion, kill bacteria, and counter the damp and cooling effects. Tacos in the U.S. that come with a flour tortilla, sour cream, refried beans, sliced lettuce, cheese and oily meat are very moistening and warming.

BEEF JERKY:

If it's spicy, beef jerky will be warming and drying. If it's salty and sweet, then it will be moistening and warming.

CORNBREAD:

It's sweet. Too much sweet causes dampness.

PEANUT BUTTER AND JELLY SANDWICH:

Peanut butter is rich and sticky. We can predict that it will be moistening and slightly warming. Jelly is very sweet so it's generally moistening.

POPCORN:

This ancient American food is light, bland and comes from fire. It will be slightly drying and cooling. Popcorn is high in antioxidant polyphenols. If you add salt and butter, it becomes warming and moistening. If you add garlic, onions or chili pepper, then it becomes drying and warming.

CLAM CHOWDER:

Rich and salty, clam chowder is cooling and moistening.

BARBECUE:

Grilled meats and vegetables are drying and warming. The types of sauces, herbs and seasoning will further change the effects on the body.

MACARONI AND CHEESE:

Warming and moistening.

GOJI BERRIES:

These berries taste sour and sweet, so we know that they are inappropriate for a cold and damp microbiome, but great for those with a warm and dry microbiome. Traditionally they are said to nourish blood.

FISH OILS:

Deep-sea fish are from a very cold and dry environment. It's dry because they are surrounded by salt water. As a result, they must retain fat and moisture. They are a rich source of oils; however, if your body is moist and cold, they are to be regarded as poison because they will continue to promote your imbalance. If your body is warmer and drier, then they become beneficial.

RAISIN BRAN:

The bran is slightly bitter and the raisins are sweet. These balance each other. Once you add sugar and milk, this cereal becomes moistening and cooling.

CHEESECAKE:

Cheesecake is incredibly rich so you can determine that it is more moistening. It is sweet so it's slightly warming.

BEER:

It depends on the beer. Some are very dark and bitter. These are more suitable for countering fat. Some are sweet, and these are more moistening. The alcohol can add heat. All alcohol will have a side effect of causing some slight food retention and killing bacteria. Beer is more suitable in a dry climate like Sumeria or Egypt where it was first invented. Bitter, warm, unpasteurized beer can help promote digestion.

TOFU:

Tofu is cooling and moistening. If you are hot and dry, then it is medicine. If you are cold and moist, it is poisonous. If you only have a little bit and counter it with pungent spices, then it balances out.

KOMBUCHA:

This is basically a fermented seaweed soup. While it may have originated in China, it is relatively unknown by the majority of the population. Its taste is acidic/sour and salty, which suggests that it is has an overall cooling effect on the gut microbiome. Research has shown antimicrobial and antioxidant activity, which would confirm it having a cooling and moistening effect on the body.

SEASONINGS

Garlic: Spicy with a warming sensation = warming and drying.

Onions: Pungent and spicy with a warming sensation = warming and drying.

Basil: Sweet and spicy = warming and drying.

Anise: Sweet and aromatic = warming and drying.

Cardamom: Spicy = warming and drying.

Cilantro: Pungent and bitter = cooling and drying.

Parsley: Pungent and slightly bitter = cooling and drying.

Cloves: Pungent with a cooling sensation = cooling and drying.

Mint: Pungent with a cooling sensation = cooling and drying.

Five-spice powder: Spicy with a warming sensation = Warming and drying.

Salt: Salt is moistening. Too much will interfere with your water metabolism.

Pepper: Spicy with a warming sensation = Warming and drying.

Chapter 7: Hot and Dry (Desert)

If you live in a warm and dry climate or if your internal microbiome has become too warm and dry:

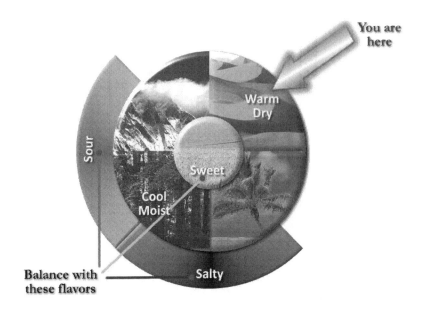

HOT AND DRY

In the hot and dry regions of the world, life is dispersed and hidden. Compared to a forest, the distance between trees is much greater. Only the hardiest plants survive. These plants adapt by holding as much moisture as possible. Because the environment is so harsh, animals burrow underground to avoid the heat by day and venture out at night. This helps them to stay cool and hydrated. Desert animals tend to grow big ears to help them cool off. By bringing blood circulation to the surface of the body, it escapes outward much easier.

The human body responds to heat by increasing circulation and by sweating. Too much heat can lead to dehydration and dryness. Heat generally manifests with red eyes, thirst, and dark urine. It is associated with skin rashes, lesions, and irritability. One of the key signs of heat is inflammation. The word inflammation literally means "on fire".

In the desert, heat can kill. The way to make yourself comfortable is to consume substances that help your internal environment stay cool. I once met a Bedouin man from Egypt. He described how his people could survive with little water:

"After a long day in the desert, a man could drink an entire lake. It is not truly his lack of water that injures him; it is the heat. We first drink a tea made of herbs. It cools the inside. After we drink even a small cup of this, we feel relief and a normal amount of water is sufficient."

Bedouin have thrived in lands that easily kill those who don't know the secrets of the desert. They have discovered how to turn their bodies into a cool garden even when the outside environment is a blistering hell. The diseases of the desert will enter the body no matter what, but once inside, they cannot survive. When Bedouin drink their herbal teas, they cool themselves by carrying an oasis within. They realize that their cravings have more to do with the regulation of moisture and temperature than anything else.

In hot, dry climates, cacti are prevalent. Cacti retain their moisture with a waxy cuticle and tend to have a bitter flavor; they can help us to retain moisture. Sunburn and constipation are symptoms of heat and dryness. You are probably already familiar with the use of aloe for sunburn or constipation.

Mexicans have traditionally eaten aloe and other cacti, which are moistening and cooling. Traditional Indian corn is also moistening and cooling with a mixture of sweet, bitter, and sour flavors. When combined with lime, corn will have a very cooling and moistening influence on the body. This makes the traditional Mexican diet perfect for a hot and arid climate.

Foods such as grapes, watermelons and dates are designed to retain moisture. Dairy products are also ideal for arid regions. Fermented yogurt with salt is a popular drink throughout Central Asia. The sour flavor makes it cooling, and the salt makes it moistening.

SIGNS OF DRY HEAT IN THE MICROBIOME

Thirst	Thirst increases with a desire for cold drinks
Skin	Dry, red, rash. Skin redness is associated with heat. Think of pimples and skin eruptions as small volcanoes. The heat is pushing its way up and out. A rash is another sign of systemic inflammation
Temperament	People with too much heat will speak in short bursts. The body is trying to force more air out on the exhalation to make the blood more alkaline. This causes people to speak as though they are shouting
Lips	Red, if the heat starts to dry up fluids, then they will get dry or chapped
Mouth	Teeth will tend to be more yellow. Possible sores on the mouth or the tongue. Bad breath, especially in the morning
Pulse	Fast
Urine	More frequently yellow
Stools	Tendency toward small sheep-like stools or constipation with an intense smell
Sleep	Heat will affect sleep. It causes people to toss and turn and have trouble getting in to a deep state of sleep
Eyes	Bloodshot eyes can indicate that the body is running a little hot
Tongue color	Red
Tongue coating	Yellow or dry without a coating

RX

If you have too much heat in your microbiome, you can cool it with plants that have a bitter flavor. These plants tend to have antibiotic, antifungal, and antiviral properties. They kill pathogenic bacteria and reduce inflammation. They also tend to move through the digestive tract faster, which further reduces body heat.

TEA

Senna Green tea   Jue Ming Zi tea

MEAT

Eat less meat   Ocean fish
(As it tends to be warming)

PLANTS

Most fruits and vegetables are cool and moistening	Cucumbers	Artichokes
	Melons	Cactus
Tofu	Cherries	Wild yams
Pine nuts	Yoghurt	Malabar tamarind
Bananas		

RECIPES FOR A HOT AND DRY MICROBIOME

FRUIT SALAD (SERVES 10)

Ingredients:

2/3 cup fresh orange juice

1/3 cup fresh lemon juice

1/3 cup packed brown sugar

1 teaspoon grated orange zest

1 teaspoon grated lemon zest

1 teaspoon vanilla extract

2 cups cubed fresh pineapple

2 cups strawberries, sliced

3 kiwi fruits, peeled and sliced

5 bananas, sliced

2 oranges, peeled and cut to size

1 cup seedless grapes

2 cups blueberries

Directions:

1. Bring orange juice, lemon juice, brown sugar, orange zest, and lemon zest to a boil in a saucepan over medium-high heat. Reduce heat to medium-low and simmer until slightly thickened, about 5 minutes. Remove from heat and stir in vanilla extract. Set aside to cool.

2. Layer the fruit in a large, clear glass bowl in this order: pineapple, strawberries, kiwi fruit, bananas, oranges, grapes, and blueberries. Pour the cooled sauce over the fruit. Cover and refrigerate for 3 to 4 hours before serving.

SPINACH AND BERRIES (SERVES 4)

Ingredients:

2 tablespoons olive oil

2 cloves garlic, slivered

2 tablespoons pine nuts

1 apple, peeled, cored and chopped

1 (10 ounce) bag fresh spinach Salt and black pepper to taste Handful of cranberries, blueberries or goji berries

Directions:

1. Heat the olive oil in a large skillet or wok over low heat. Add the garlic, pine nuts, and apple; cook until the nuts and garlic are golden and the apple is just soft, 3 to 5 minutes.

2. Increase the heat to medium, and add the spinach to the skillet. Stir and cook another 2 to 3 minutes. Season with salt and pepper to taste.

WATERMELON

Slice and enjoy.

SALMON WITH PINE NUTS

Ingredients:

4 salmon fillets, about 1 1/2 pounds

1/4 cup pine nuts, toasted

1/4 cup berries Salt and pepper to taste

Olive oil, for finishing

2 large handfuls mixed herbs such as parsley, dill, or chervil

2 bunches Swiss chard (or kale), stemmed and torn into small pieces

Directions:

1. Bring 1 inch of water to boil in the bottom of two pots fitted with a steamer insert. Season the salmon fillets liberally with salt and pepper. Lay the mixed herbs in the bottom of the steamer basket and arrange the fillets on top of it. Cover the pot and steam until the salmon just begins to flake, about ten minutes.

2. When the salmon is halfway cooked, add the chard (or kale) to the second pot. Steam until tender, about 5 minutes. Sprinkle with salt and toss well to combine.

3. Divide the kale between four plates, then transfer the fillets on top. Garnish with the pine nuts and berries,

and drizzle the whole dish with olive oil. Serve with sea salt as needed.

TZATZIKI SAUCE

Ingredients:

1 pound of cucumbers, ends (6 "baby" cucumbers)

4 cloves of garlic, minced fine removed and sliced lengthwise

1 large handful of dill, minced

Juice of one lemon

2 cups of strained yogurt (Greek or otherwise)

Directions:

1. With a teaspoon, scoop out the seeds of the cucumbers. You should be left with a neat half-moon shape. Slice them thin, but not paper-thin – they should still have some crunch.

2. Add the cucumbers to a mixing bowl along with the rest of the ingredients. Taste for acid and seasoning,

then either serve or (preferably) cover and let sit in the refrigerator for a few hours.

Chapter 8: Hot and Moist (Tropical)

If you live in a moist and warm environment, or if your internal microbiome has become too tropical:

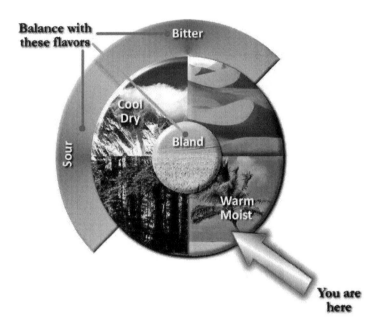

HOT AND MOIST

The rainforest hums. Tiny feet pitter-patter over wet leaves. In the warm nights animals sing erotic serenades. Life is abundant and competition is fierce. Trees race to reach the canopy, choking out their competition. The fallen quickly rot and rejoin the soil. These hot, wet climates host most of Earth's species. This rivalry inspires living things to adorn themselves with bright colors. They spread seeds in sweet fruit. They display beauty in movement, color and sound. They protect themselves with piercing points and with poison. This is where you can find some of the most chemically active plants and animals. You can also find an intensity of decay.

Leaves spread out evenly across a forest floor will turn into mulch at a consistent rate. If you rake those same leaves into a pile and cover them to retain moisture, they will get hot from all the microbial activity. In some instances, they can get so hot that they catch fire.

Something similar can happen inside the human body. In Chinese medicine, this is called "Damp Fire". When people have food retention, it leaves piles of debris behind. When your gut gets too moist and compacted, it creates conditions similar to a compost fire. While people don't tend to catch fire, they can get low-grade fever and chronic inflammation that is associated with a host of chronic diseases.

Hot and humid climates grow mold. To prevent your body from getting a fungal overgrowth, you need to improve water metabolism. When water sits in the space outside of your cells at 98.6 degrees Fahrenheit, pathogenic microbiota begin to proliferate. Your body will try to kill them off through your inflammatory response. This can give you a low-grade fever of unknown origin. Many people with a chronic low fever are actually in a slow state of composting and the body is fighting in vain to stop it.

Although exercise can help, the body's sodium potassium pumps are already overloaded, so exercise will tend to make people feel tired. The increased inflammatory reaction in the body also makes it easier for joints to ache. This further immobilizes people and keeps them from exercising. The majority of modern people have an excess of dampness and heat which can contribute to type 2 fibromyalgia pain.

SIGNS OF DAMP HEAT IN THE MICROBIOME	
Thirst	Feeling dry, but not having a desire to drink liquid or forgetting to drink enough water
Teeth	Yellow tint
Ears	Increased earwax
Discharge	Yellow
Skin	Weeping rashes, acne on the insides of the legs, and/or edema
Sleep	Sleep obstruction, snoring, or sleep apnea
Eyes	In severe cases there is a yellowish tint
Urine	Yellow, sandy or frothy
Stools	Tendency toward sloppy or sticky stools
Temperament	Tired, lethargic
Fungal infections	Tendency to get fungal infections. These frequently manifest as toenail fungus, sinus infections, yeast infections, jock itch, athletes foot, chronic mucus, thrush, etc.
Tongue color	Red or pale depending on the degree of inflammation
Tongue coating	Thick yellow coating

DRAIN THE SWAMP

The stagnant water of a swamp is a good place to find alligators and mosquitoes. If you live in a swamp and choose not to get eaten alive, you have two choices: You can either poison the water, or drain the swamp. If you poison the water, the alligators may swim away for a while and the mosquitoes will die, but eventually both will return when the bleach wears off. If you drain the swamp, it will change the landscape into grassland. The alligators will either have to move on or they will die. The mosquito eggs will also die if they don't get enough moisture. When it comes to dampness and heat in the body, the most important strategy is to drain off the extra water.

RX

Reduce water retention: Use bitter and bland foods to increase urination. To lend flavor, use pungent foods to increase sweating and further dry the body.

GENERAL

Enjoy fewer salty, sour, and sweet foods.

Instead, introduce more foods which are bitter, sour and slightly pungent.

Examples: Ginger, garlic, kimchi, sauerkraut

EXERCISES

Activities that increase sweating, urination, and defecation can be beneficial. Sauna, getting appropriate sunlight, and stomach massage.

MEAT

Think of things that live in dirty water. These creatures have the chemical structures to deal with water retention and microbes. Meat is generally to be avoided when the microbiome becomes too hot as it tends to be warming.

Freshwater fish   Frogs   Alligator

PLANTS

Freshwater aquatic plants have incredible water transport mechanisms to stay dry and avoid rotting. If you don't have these, use other vegetables and add the appropriate spices.

Watercress	Lotus	Pearl barley
Cattails	Water chestnut	Job's tears
Rice	Taro	Rye
Water pepper	Chinese water chestnut	Mushrooms
Water spinach		Bitter melon
Wasabi	Bitter green	Winter melon

MUSHROOMS

Mushrooms are among the more palatable bitter foods. They are also some of the most useful for maintaining a balanced microbiome. Mushrooms break things down. That is what they do for a living. Not just leftovers in the fridge, but toxic waste, oil sludge and radioactive materials. Mushrooms and fungi are being used to repair damaged ecosystems and renew polluted environments through a process called mycoremediation. World-renowned mycologist Paul Stamets explains it like this: "Fungi recycle plants after they die and transform them into rich soil. If not for mushrooms and fungi, the Earth would be buried in several feet of debris and life on the planet would soon disappear."

Remember that your internal microbiome is not so different from our external one. This is good news because you are constantly eating poison. It's really okay. Everything has a little poison and it's not a big deal if you keep it balanced. Mushrooms break down accumulations of food and act as prebiotics. By keeping the gut stocked with beneficial bacteria, they increase competition in the gut, making it difficult for food and airborne allergens to disrupt our internal ecosystem.

Mushrooms help to lower cholesterol and fat. Sundried mushrooms are also excellent sources of vitamin D. Mushrooms contain very little, if any, vitamin D2 but are abundant in ergosterol, which can be converted into vitamin D2 by ultraviolet (UV) radiation.

RECIPES FOR A HOT AND MOIST MICROBIOME

JOB'S TEARS PORRIDGE (SERVES 2)

Ingredients:

2 oz. (55g) Job's tears

3–5 pieces rock sugar

3–5 cups of water

Directions:

1. Put Job's tears and water into a saucepan, and bring quickly to a boil. Reduce heat; simmer for 30 minutes until Job's tears become soft.

2. Add rock sugar and stir.

3. Serve warm.

MUSHROOM ROMAINE HEART (SERVES 2)

Ingredients:

1 romaine heart, torn into pieces

8 oz. fresh shiitake mushrooms, sliced

1/4 teaspoon salt

2 tablespoons vegetable oil

Directions:

1. Heat the oil in a pan over medium heat.

2. Add shiitake mushrooms and stir for 1 minute.

3. Add romaine heart and stir until leaves are soft.

4. Add salt and mix well. Serve warm.

For Severe Damp Heat

MUNG BEAN JOB'S TEARS GRUEL (SERVES 2)

Ingredients:

2 oz. (55g) mung beans

1 oz. (30g) Job's tears

4 oz. (110g) white rice

8–10 cups of water

Directions:

1. Put mung beans and Job's tears in water. Bring to a boil.

2. Add rice. Bring back to a boil and turn down the heat to simmer. Stir from time to time.

3. Simmer for 30 minutes or until it forms a gruel.

4. Serve warm.

Chapter 9: Cold

Cold is the relative absence of metabolism. Antibiotics, bitter herbs, ice water, sedentary behavior and foods served at cooler temperatures will all slow down the metabolism of your microbiome. If your body thinks you are cold, it will try to dress you in a layer of fat for warmth. This is why people feel hungrier as autumn begins. Feeling cold signals ghrelin. This hormone regulates hunger as well as the rate of energy expenditure. If food is scarce or the weather is cold it reduces hunger and makes people sleepy. The body is responding to signals produced by experiencing darkness and cold.

Eating triggers metabolic activity, which raises the level of heat in your body. If your body feels cold, it signals you to eat for short-term warmth and then sends signals for long-term appetite so that you store fat and have insulation in the long run.

SEDENTARY WORLD

In today's sedentary world, we are much colder metabolically than we have ever been. Few of us run to work or spend the day walking up hills as we forage for food.

Sedentary behavior can make people cooler than they otherwise would be with sufficient exercise. The amount people eat often has more to do with temperature regulation than it does with meeting the body's nutritional requirements.

RAW FOOD

Generally speaking, raw food is cold. It requires quite a bit of energy to warm and "cook" the food inside of our body.

Raw food can be a great source of sustenance and sometimes people don't have the luxury of cooking. If you look at how raw foods are eaten around the world, you will find that they are warmed with herbs, alcohol or lifestyle adaptation.

Sushi and sashimi are Japanese foods with varying amounts of raw fish. They are traditionally eaten with pickled ginger and wasabi, which is incredibly pungent. The wasabi goes right up the nose and clears the sinuses. The fish is cold and dense, while the wasabi and ginger is expansive and moving. When sweet and pungent flavors combine, they create a warming effect. When this is combined with rice wine, it further acts to warm the raw fish and cold rice.

When we visit our brother-in-law in the Tibetan plateau, we sometimes eat raw frozen yak. We mix it with garlic and a chili pepper sauce. The chili pepper sauce and the garlic will kill anything growing on the yak and you wash it all down with a kind of fermented grain liquor. The combination of spices and alcohol helps to "warm" the frozen food.

SIGNS OF COLD IN THE MICROBIOME	
Thirst	Low thirst. Desire for warm drinks
Skin	White or pale because the blood is stored in the internal organs
Temperature	Cold limbs, easily chilled, dislike of wind or cold weather
Emotions	More tired or lethargic
Lips	Pale
Mouth	If the body becomes too cold, the mouth may develop thrush
Pulse	Slow
Urine	Frequent and clear
Stools	Tendency toward diarrhea, infrequent stools, or stools with undigested food
Tongue color	Pale
Tongue coating	White
Tongue color	Red or pale depending on the degree of inflammation
Tongue coating	Thick yellow coating

DITCH THE ICE

If you have ever cleaned an oily pan, you know that fat becomes a solid quickly when it cools and is very difficult to clean. When you eat the oils found in food and follow it with an iced drink, the fats congeal. Think of cold butter coming out of the freezer and then imagine that you have to break it down to the molecular level. Now imagine that you have melted butter. Which do you think will be easier? When foods are warm, they dissolve easily because the molecules are moving faster. Heat expands and cold contracts. It is a basic phenomenon of nature.

Iced drinks are largely poisonous for sedentary people with relatively cool microbiomes. It isn't the temperature itself that is poisonous; it is the compost heap it creates when food doesn't get broken down and starts to decay inside of you. Knowing the right temperature for your microbiome is easy. If your tongue is fat or has a thick coating, then use warmer liquids and foods. If your tongue is fine and you are feeling strong to the point that you would feel comfortable pouring something of the same temperature on top of your head, then it is probably fine to drink.

Imagine icing your eyes before attempting to take a vision

test. You could expect that the changes in blood circulation would cause some visual disturbances. Just as your eyes cannot see well without blood, your digestive organs cannot function well without proper blood circulation.

RAW VEGETABLES

You may have heard that raw vegetables will lose their vitamins if they are cooked. This information is nice, but it is useless. It doesn't matter whatsoever how many vitamins are in food when it rests on your table. It only matters how much you can actually eat and absorb. There are also practical limitations to the amount of vegetables you can actually eat when you have them raw. If you were to find a giant salad bowl like the kind used at large receptions, you would have a good idea of the amount of vegetables you should be eating in a single day. Of course, eating that many raw vegetables without constant physical exercise wouldn't be appetizing. On the other hand, if you were to fry up all of these same vegetables in garlic and ginger, you could finish this in a single meal. This is because it is physically easier to eat.

Plants don't actually want to be eaten. You can't blame them. They come with tiny barbs, hairs and poisons to keep themselves off of the menu. Cooking vegetables helps to break down these defenses and neutralize poisons. Cooking makes vegetables easier to chew and it shrinks the vegetables considerably. There are times when raw vegetables are just fine. It's conditional on how your body is responding to the outside environment. If you have more heat, then raw vegetables are probably fine. If you are feeling cold, cook them first and add some spices.

Chapter 10: Cold and Dry (Arctic Microbiome)

If you live in a cold, dry region or if your internal microbiome has become cold and dry:

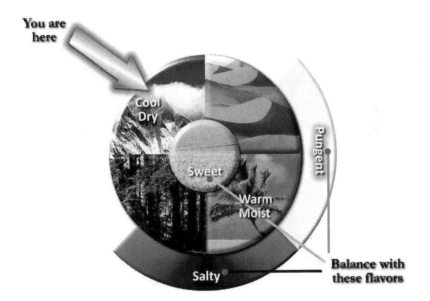

COLD AND DRY

The cold, dry air of the Arctic causes life to slow to a crawl. The slow decay and sparse plant life contributes to poor soil quality. Plant life grows briefly in summer and then must prepare for the icy hibernation of winter. Every animal in this environment must adapt. They insulate themselves in fat and burrow underground to create warmer microclimates.

SIGNS OF COLD DRYNESS IN THE MICROBIOME	
Thirst	Desire for warm drinks
Skin	White, patchy, and dry
Temperature	Cold limbs, easily chilled, dislike of wind or cold weather
Emotions	Tired or lethargic
Lips	Tendency toward pale and chapped lips
Mouth	If the body becomes too cold, the mouth may develop thrush
Pulse	Slow
Urine	Frequent and clear
Stools	Tendency toward diarrhea with undigested stools
Tongue color	Pale
Tongue coating	White

In the Arctic, life itself seems to escape with every breath. The air pulls water and heat out of your skin. In the Arctic, people need to stay warm and moist. As northern peoples eat nutritionally dense foods, it provides more metabolic heat. It creates a tropical greenhouse inside, serving as a climate barrier against the frigid landscape. To help maintain this barrier they use pungent foods such as leeks, garlic or hard liquor to maintain warmth. Where pungent foods are scarce, sweat baths achieve similar effects. Smokehouses and saunas can be found throughout the Arctic Circle from Scandinavia to Alaska. These saunas provide a climate barrier and also help people generate nitric oxide, which helps them to maintain gut balance. When people have free circulating nitric oxide, then cold exposure can stimulate their body to begin turning fat into heat and usable energy. Without developing nitric oxide production through hard physical work or saunas and having cold exposure, this rich diet can lead to gut dysbiosis, and fibromyalgia.

RX

Spices

Root vegetables such as ginger, garlic and salt

MEATS

Animals from cold climates or high altitudes. Reindeer, duck, seal, walrus, yak, whale, fatty and nutrient-dense foods, warming foods

PLANTS

Use fewer fruits. Enjoy leeks, radishes and other warming plants.

RECIPES FOR A COLD AND DRY MICROBIOME

BEEF AND CARROTS (SERVES 2)

Ingredients:

3 pounds beef, cut into chunks

2 tablespoons soy sauce

Salt and pepper to taste

4 carrots, cut into chunks

2 tablespoons vegetable oil

5 pieces garlic, 2 sliced, 3

3 cups chicken broth (or whole water)

3 pieces ginger, sliced

1 egg white, whipped

3 pieces spring onion, chopped

Directions:

1. Marinate beef with sliced garlic, ginger, soy sauce and egg white for 1 hour.

2. Heat vegetable oil in a pan over medium-high heat until hot. Add marinated beef. Stir until the beef surface is no longer bloody.

3. Add chicken broth and cover the pan with a lid. Turn down to low medium-low heat when the broth is boiled. Cook until the beef is about fork-tender.

4. Add carrots. Cook until the carrots are soft. Season with salt and pepper to taste. Turn off the heat.

5. Sprinkle the spring onion on the dish and serve warm.

Chapter 11: Cold and Moist (Temperate Rainforest Microbiome)

If you live in a moist and cool region or if your internal microbiome has become too moist and cool:

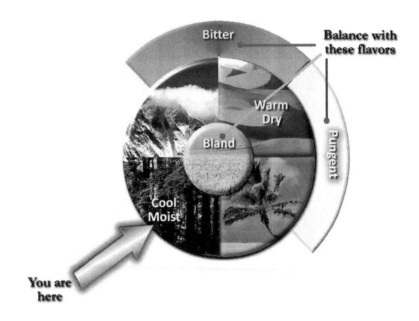

COLD AND MOIST

The animals in a temperate forest sing, but not with the complexity of their tropical cousins. The flowers bloom and fruits ripen, but more modestly than their tropical counterparts. Cool weather slows the collective metabolism.

There is less density of life and less competition than the tropics.

There are certainly areas of the body that should be swampy, but when this extends into areas which are meant to be dry, it creates problems. Sedentary living reduces fluid metabolism. This can lead to water retention. When the internal microbiome becomes cold and damp, it overloads your water transport mechanisms. It doesn't matter how much water you are drinking. What is important is that your body is distributing all of the water you absorb.

Any fluid left behind makes your body soggy. This can cause your body to begin slowly rotting like an old tree in the forest.

SIGNS OF COLD DAMPNESS IN THE MICROBIOME	
Thirst	When people have dampness, they will typically lose their sense of thirst and have to remind themselves to drink water
Urine	Clear and frothy, possibly cloudy
Stools	Tendency toward sloppy or sticky stools
Discharge	White
Fungal infections	Tendency to get fungal infections: Toenail fungus, sinus infections, yeast infections, jock itch, athletes foot, chronic mucus, thrush
Skin	Weeping rashes, acne on the insides of the legs, edema
Sleep	Sleep obstruction, snoring, or sleep apnea
Temperament	Tired, lethargic
Tongue color	Pale
Tongue shape	Fat with marks on the side where the tongue is pushing into the teeth. This shows reduced water metabolism and increased extracellular fluid
Tongue coating	Possibly with a thick white coating

COLD AND DRY VS. COLD AND DAMP:

The key point to observe is urine production. With cold damp, there is less urination and it tends to be frothy. With pure cold, there is a desire to urinate often and the urine tends to be clear and scanty. Cold and damp tends to come with fungal infections. The tongue coating in both cold and cold damp can be white, but with dampness the tongue coating tends to be thicker. When the body is cold and dry you see signs of dry skin and mucus membranes, and poor skin luster.

RX

Dry out by increasing sweating, urination and defecation

GENERAL

Sauna, getting appropriate sunlight, and stomach massage are all ideal.

SPICES

Dry the water by warming the body Sichuan peppercorn

Ginger Pepper Chili peppers Garlic Cumin Kimchi

TEA

Use teas which are slightly spicy and known for settling the stomach.

Pu-er tea   Black tea   Ginger tea

MEATS

Think of things that live in a forest. These creatures have the chemical structure to deal with the cold and damp climate.

River fish   Elk   Pheasant

Deer   Beef   Chicken

PLANTS

Freshwater aquatic plants are the best. They must have incredible water transport mechanisms to stay dry and avoid rotting. If you don't have these, use other vegetables and add the appropriate spices.

Watercress	Lotus	Pearl barley
Cattails	Water chestnut	Job's tears
Rice	Taro	Rye
Water pepper	Chinese water chestnut	
Water spinach		
Wasabi	Bitter green vegetables	

HERBAL PROFILE: SICHUAN PEPPERCORNS

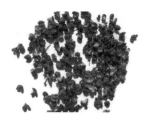

Sichuan peppercorns, or "hua jiao", contain a flavor called "ma la" which means that it is numbing and spicy. When you eat it, it provides a numbing and tingly feeling around the lips. This spice is used in damp climates to strongly warm and dry the body. It is highly antifungal and kills certain parasites. It is anti-inflammatory and has been shown to increase pain threshold.

Add this simple spice to both meat and vegetable dishes to counter the effects of oil and help counter the oil. You can find it in most Asian grocery stores. If there is a language barrier, simply show them this: "花椒". This spice is useful for warming the body, and reducing the pain of fibromyalgia by addressing type 2 and type 8 fibromyalgia pain.

HERBAL PROFILE: CHILI PEPPERS

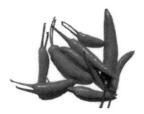

Chili peppers are warm, spicy and pungent. They can help warm a cool microbiome and help to burn away fat. They have anti-inflammatory and painkilling effects on the body, which can help those with chronic pain enjoy greater mobility.

RECIPES FOR A COLD AND MOIST MICROBIOME

FOUR SEASON BEANS (SERVES 3–4)

Ingredients:

1 lb. green beans, ends cut

3–4 pieces garlic, minced off, cut into half

2 teaspoons Sichuan

1–2 pieces dry red peppercorn chili pepper, chopped

3 tablespoons vegetable oil (optional)

1/4 teaspoon salt

1 piece fresh ginger, minced

Directions:

1. Heat vegetable oil in a frying pan over medium-low heat. Add garlic, ginger and chili pepper to the oil and sauté.

2. Add green beans and keep stirring till the skin of

green beans starts to shrink.

3. Turn off the heat. Add 1/4 teaspoon of salt and stir evenly.

4. Serve warm.

To make it warmer and more drying, add more Sichuan peppercorns.

Chapter 12: Secrets of Microbiome Mastery

1. When you cook two foods together, you create something new.

The chemical structures in food change depending on how they are cooked and what they are cooked with. This is why considering the individual properties of food is of little use in considering the overall effect of a cooked meal.

2. Depending on what you eat, it may influence the absorption of other foods

This happens due to changes in gastric pH balance as well as the chemical interaction of other substances you have recently ingested.

3. By changing the ratio of food flavors, you can control the overall effects of the meal

The ratio of flavors will alter the effects on the body. If you have a food that is 60 percent warming and drying and mix it with a food that is 40 percent cooling and moistening, then the overall effect will be slightly warming and drying. If you eat an entire block of cheese and attempt to balance it with some bitter parsley, it won't remotely help keep you from becoming too damp. The cheese will overpower the parsley. On the other hand, if you were to combine some rye crackers, mushrooms and Pu-er tea with a thin slice of cheese, then the moistening effect of the cheese would be negligible because the overall effect of the meal would be to dry the body.

4. The reverse assistant

The idea of the reverse assistant is to use a flavor with the opposite effect to ensure that you never tip too far in one direction. If your microbiome is cold and you want to warm it, go ahead and add warming foods, but always add something which is cooling to ensure that you don't go too far.

5. Combining safe foods can create poison

When people don't understand how to combine flavors and balance their microbiome, they often combine perfectly good foods in ways that are ultimately destructive.

One of the primary ways people do this is by using ineffective methods of food preparation. If you take a number of fruits and vegetables, remove the pulp and mix them together with ice and blend, you create a smoothie. You don't have a fruit salad. Instead you basically have a milkshake. It doesn't matter how many vitamins get thrown into the mix – once it's a smoothie, it's no longer the sum of its parts. Your body is going to receive a cold and clumpy helping of sugar. This can slow gut metabolism and overload your pancreas. What is left is a sludge. If you are enjoying a 20-mile run after the smoothie, then your body heat and metabolism will eventually work it all out, but this way of eating makes your body have to work overtime to accomplish its basic functions.

In this case, removing the pulp changes the timing of sugar release. It can make very healthy foods into something hard for the body to handle. Through improper processing, it is easy to turn safe and healthy foods into something that is toxic once it's inside your system.

Even with proper food preparation, there are some foods that aren't suitable together. This isn't always due to flavor, but rather experience from people who share a similar microbiome.

In China, they have the following food combining prohibitions. I'm not sure if this will affect every population the same way as microbiota can vary depending on people's environment and dietary habits.

Dates + Spring onion or fish: may cause indigestion

Celery + Chrysanthemum: may cause vomiting

Tomato + Hairy crab (aka Chinese mitten crab): may cause diarrhea

Onion + Honey: may cause eye discomfort

Pumpkin/Squash + Shrimp: may cause diarrhea

It's hard to say whether these food combinations are always toxic for every race and ethnicity on the planet, but if a certain food combination wrecks your insides, then it may be good information to pass on to your family.

6. One food can be used to counter the poisons in another

Chinese herbs are traditionally paired so that they

maximize the benefits while cancelling out side effects. You can use this same idea in cooking. Substances such as ginger can be used to reduce the effects of plant-based poisons. When you eat fish, you will encounter some toxicity. People cook with ginger both to warm the stomach and counter the effects of poison.

Fish often contain heavy metals. It's always been this way and it's okay. Seaweed and certain types of microbiota can help scavenge the heavy metals and reduce toxicity in the body.

Sichuan province in China has some of the hottest, oiliest food on the planet. The spices serve to kill off the fungi that tend to get into people and contribute to rheumatoid arthritis. The locals become accustomed to having incredible levels of spice throughout the course of their lives. For people from other places, the extreme levels of oil and spices in Sichuanese cuisine can literally hospitalize them.

If this toxic level of spice is too potent, Sichuanese people add another poison to balance things out, using grain alcohol or vinegar to ameliorate the spice. The rice liquor alone is severely potent at over 50 percent alcohol. This can do quite a bit of damage on its own because of the antibacterial effects it will have on your gut flora.

By having the two together, you can enjoy extreme levels of spice and liquor while limiting the side effects of both. Distilled alcohol is acidic, and the chili peppers are basic. While they have opposite functions, they ameliorate each other's side effects.

7. Neutralizing food

Tofu is cold and moistening. To prevent it from being too cold, many Chinese people balance it by soaking the tofu in chili peppers and Sichuan peppercorns, making the overall flavor pungent and warming. This is a very different thing from forming tofu into the shape of a turkey and having it with vegan gravy. The Chinese dish is relatively balanced. By contrast, the North American rendition of tofu is extremely cold and moistening. When adding an exotic food to your diet, always consider cultural context.

In the Middle East and the Mediterranean, people enjoy lamb. Unfortunately, lamb is pungent and warming. These kinds of foods can make it very easy to get too hot in warm weather. To avoid this they combine the lamb with cooling yoghurt or mint to balance the meal.

In Germany, cooler weather inspired people to eat dense foods such as meats, fats and heavy starches. The mixture of salty and pungent foods creates a damp and warm microbiome. To prevent it from going too far, they traditionally enjoyed cooling sauerkraut, which is sour and bitter. They also drank bitter beer and digestive liqueurs. These flavors served to balance the meal and promote healthy digestion.

8. Adjusting to reality

A friend may offer you a cheese casserole. This is sticky and rich, so you can determine that it will probably have a moistening effect on your body. If your body is already too soggy and cold, then the food is potentially poisonous to your microbiome. We do not recommend that you go into a rant on how it is unhealthy. This would be far more damaging socially and emotionally than eating a bit of cheese. Instead, counter the moisture by adding pepper, which is dry and warming. It might not be enough, but it's a step in the right direction. If you also enjoy wine or an herbal digestive liquor with the meal, it can help to break down the cheese. If you add something with fiber that is bitter, such as mushrooms, then you can ameliorate the side effects of the food. True microbiome mastery isn't about perfection, but about doing the best with what you have and flexibly adapting. It's better to be happy with what you have and to be good company than to be picky about your food and cause undue social tension. As you learn to bring balance to your gut you will have more flexibility to enjoy inappropriate foods without consequence.

LEAVE SOME SPACE

Eat until you are about 80 percent full. If you can't feel how full you are, then you need to slow down and pay attention.

EAT SLOWLY

Even if you can't eat the best foods for the right occasions, you can still find balance by simply taking it slowly and giving your body time to work things out. Think of adding flour into a mixer. If you add a lot of flour at once, it gets clumpy. It takes more effort to churn. If you add the flour gradually, it mixes evenly. Eating slowly helps your body to detect what you are eating and produce the right enzymes and digestive juices to efficiently digest your meal. It also allows your food to get enough saliva.

THE MOST PRECIOUS PILL

A river runs through your internal garden. This river is born of six salivary wells. The seventh cranial nerve activates three pairs of salivary glands, which act as tributaries filling the pool of the mouth. Within this pool, the saliva begins restoring order, cleaning your teeth, and starting the digestive process. As you swallow, it flows like a river, nourishing your enteric garden and restoring the balance of microbial life.

Classical Chinese texts go into great detail on the cultivation of saliva. It is called golden dew, elixir of life, or jade juice. It is considered to be a magic pill for longevity. If you find that hard to swallow, consider that saliva is far more than something to spit upon your enemies.

Saliva contains an important mix of electrolytes, enzymes, immunoglobulins, and other factors important for oral and digestive health. It increases your body's metabolism and helps you to fight off disease. One component of saliva, amylase, helps to break down sugars. Many people have low levels of this enzyme. This is important because if you have enough amylase and are using it properly, you can obtain the sugar you need and use it efficiently. Digestive enzymes such as amylase are manufactured in the pancreas. The quality of those enzymes determines how well you can break down and use food. These enzymes also break down slimy biofilms in the body that guard pathogenic bacteria.

Saliva is very healing. It can encourage skin growth and speeds blood clotting. This is why animals lick their wounds.

When it comes to gardening your biome of microbiota, saliva does most of the work. It prevents colonization by disease-causing microorganisms by changing their growing conditions. This is an elegant way to detour even the most malevolent microbes. For those that don't take the hint, your saliva has a backup plan. It contains a variety of proteins with antibacterial and antiviral properties. Saliva contains lysozyme, which can dissolve unwelcome bacteria. It can also starve bacteria of iron using lactoferrin, which hoards the available iron. It starves bacteria such as strep, which would be perfectly happy to give you a sore throat.

Your saliva flows at different rates throughout the day. With respect to this, you should pay close attention to the timing of meals, being as consistent as possible and following natural cycles for optimum health. Saliva slows to a crawl at night and is more active by day. This is one reason why eating at night is less efficient. Another way you can interfere with saliva is by washing it away, which can affect our ability to properly absorb nutrition.

EXERCISE: CULTIVATING SALIVA

1. Begin by gathering saliva for 5 breaths, circling the tongue around your teeth 9 times each way.

2. Keep collecting it and breathe deeply. As the saliva collects it will begin to clean your teeth.

3. Begin gently tapping your teeth together to increase salivary production.

4. Swallow the saliva. Visualize the saliva sinking. Feel it through the digestive tract as it reaches your stomach. Picture it bringing order to your gut garden and feel

the changes it makes. Look inward and feel how much the stomach is moving. Try to visualize the nerves around the stomach to give yourself an approximate picture. Feel your gut's enteric nervous system as your saliva begins to garden your internal microbiome.

COMPLEX PATTERNS

You can feel cold on the inside and feel hot to the touch. You can also have a hot microbiome and yet feel cold. It can be confusing, but this is why you can never go by a single symptom. Feeling cold or hot is only one indication. You must also consider appetite, urine, stools, sleep and other signs to get an idea of how your system is tipping. If you have a seemingly hot microbiome, yet feel cold or have strange sensations such as heat in the upper body or cold below, it's time to see a Chinese medical professional to get it sorted out.

ATTEMPTING PERFECTION

Your internal balance is always tipping. This flux is part of life. As long as you keep it from getting too far out of bounds, it's really easy to maintain. In fact, it's important to take a relaxed attitude about it. It is a mistake to do everything correctly with this approach. If you get it above 75 percent right, it's good enough. Going too far in one direction can quickly become overcorrection and leads to further extremes. Being too strict about diet can raise anxiety. People understand the toxicity of smoking, and they know that donuts are not the healthiest thing to eat, yet they underestimate the toxicity of anxiety and obsession. These feelings release hormones which interfere with digestion. Once more, being too strict is a poor way to keep balance. You can't walk a tightrope logically – it's something you get a feeling for. By keeping the legs soft and the body aligned and relaxed, you can do a better job. The same is true of diet. You can use the general principles as a guideline, but attempting to be perfect is not the best way to maintain your natural balance.

GRADUAL CHANGES

Begin by using a greater range of flavors and colors in your meals. This will increase your microbial biodiversity. As you get used to this you can begin to discover the effect different flavors have on your body. If you feel cold and damp, increase pungent, bland and bitter foods, but stay at around 60–75 percent of the flavors in the meal. If your internal microbiome is too cold and damp, using lots of garlic and onions can warm it, but you don't want to go overboard. If you suddenly go to an extreme with warming and drying foods, you can expect constipation, poor sleep and stomach upset. Make sure that change comes slowly and comfortably and that there is still a healthy mix of colors and flavors.

MAKING THE BEST OF WHAT YOU HAVE

Adapting to environmental change has been the core thread of human history.

Your ancestors endured environmental radiation, poisonous plants and toxic volcanic fumes, and yet here you are. Imperfection is perfectly acceptable. Your body only requires that you do your best to keep things in balance. Sometimes you eat things that are less than ideal. You take in preservatives, poisons and toxic radiation. That is okay. With the principles outlined in this book you can make the best of even the worst foods and maintain internal harmony.

Chapter 13: Useful Tools
THE POWER OF TEA

Lu Tong, a Chinese poet, wrote, "Seven bowls of tea bring seven advantages: one, it promotes the production of body fluids and quenches thirst; two, it refreshes the mind; three, it helps digestion; four, it induces sweating to relieve the common cold; five, it helps fat people reduce weight; six, it activates thinking and strengthens memory; and seven, it ensures longevity."

Assuming that Lu Tong was correct, the only reason the tea might actually affect all of these properties, from treating a common cold to fat reduction and increased memory, is if tea had a special influence on gut microbiota.

Fibrokalm Tea

Some teas are designed to protect the digestive system from the influences of stress. One such tea, "Xiao Yao San", was first described in *Prescriptions of the Imperial Pharmacy During the Great Age of Peace* in 1107AD. Today, Xiao Yao San is one of the most commonly used Chinese medicines in Asia, well regarded both for its safety and efficacy[6]. Xiao Yao San is designed to help smooth the flow of qi in the body. Research has shown that it can lower levels of circulating nitric oxide, making it function similarly to acupuncture to reduce nitric oxide in order to smooth the overall flow.

Depending on the dosage, it is frequently used for anxiety, dyspepsia, acne, menstrual disorders, sleep disorders, jet lag, depression, obesity and fibromyalgia. Because it acts on regulatory centers, it neither excites nor depresses in the absolute sense, but it has the ability to do both.

Research has shown that it can reduce pain, stress, anxiety, and appetite. It even works as well as antidepressant medications for depression. It has direct regulatory effects on the hypothalamus, nervous, endocrine, and immune systems. These systems work together to regulate mood and improve neuroplasticity. This helps the brain to reorganize itself and form new connections. It has also been shown to be highly effective for fibromyalgia pain.

PICKLED VEGETABLES

---

[6] *Increase β-endorphin, which acts on opioid receptors and lowers corticotropin releasing factor1 (CRF-1).*

Pickled vegetables are great for maintaining a healthy microbiome. The wider the variety of vegetables that you pickle, the more diverse your microbiota will become. Kimchi is Korea's national food. This comes with good reason: these pickled foods are packed with probiotics, making it easy to keep a well-functioning microbiome. Kimchi can reduce gas and has been shown to inhibit appetite. Lactobacillus in pickled vegetables can help stabilize blood sugar. Kimchi is rich in vitamins and has lactic acid, which has demonstrated anti-obesity effects in animal studies. If you haven't found yourself to be a fan of dill pickles, pick up some kimchi at the grocery store. Pickling is easy to do at home and there are pickling traditions from all over the world. Pick one.

TO RECAP

-To warm and moisten the microbiome, use mostly pungent, sweet, rich and oily foods.

-To warm and dry: Use more pungent, bland and bitter foods.

-To cool and moisten: Use sour, salty and sweet foods.

-To cool and dry: Use bitter, sour and bland foods.

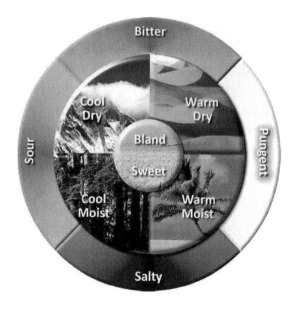

Part II

Chapter 14: The Breath of the Universe

"And He breathed into his nostrils the breath of life, and the man became a living being."

—*Genesis 2:7*

The gases in the universe form a living breath. The sun is a burning ball of gas. Hydrogen and oxygen combine to form droplets of water, which fall to Earth as rain. In a flash of lighting, nitrogen descends to Earth. As this breath of the heavens mixes with soil, the land becomes a living thing.

The gases in the heavens descend to the Earth, allowing life to thrive. As the winds blow over the landscape, microbiota in the soil rise up on vapors into the atmosphere. Sometimes when the light is just so, you can see the fullness of the air.

I was maybe six years old when it first dawned on me that the air wasn't empty. In the morning light, sunbeams shone through an old window. I could see the dust floating and swirling in imperceptible currents. It seemed at once like an undulating ocean or the swirling of the cosmos.

If you could see microbiota the way I first saw dust, the entire world would seem to be one continuous mass of life spanning from the stratosphere to subterranean caves and even your most hidden veins. They travel on currents of gas as fish swim in streams. They are not only sustained by these gases; they change them.

Everything living has a complex interaction with the gases that sustain their existence. They influence the atmosphere and also contribute to its changes. Our own atmosphere has been anything but static over the ages. In the past, bacteria changed the entire atmosphere and caused a mass extinction. At one time, oxygen was deadly to most life on Earth. There was one small bacterium which used the sun's energy and expelled oxygen as a waste product. As the Earth's balance shifted, these cyanobacteria began to proliferate. They produced so much oxygen that they contributed to destroying most life on Earth. In the new atmosphere, everything needed to tolerate oxygen or it would die. Oxygen-loving creatures thrived and continue to do so now.

Depending on the amount of phytoplankton in the oceans and forest cover on land, oxygen levels on Earth have been as high as 35 percent. Today we enjoy around 20 percent oxygen saturation. In the forest, plants respire. Mushrooms create their own microclimate and spread spores by releasing water vapor to cool the air around them and create tiny wind currents. From the flapping of a butterfly's wing to the collective exhalation of the Amazon rainforest, everything interacts with the air. Where gases go, life follows.

The scent before a rain isn't the scent of water, but rather the blooming mold within the water particles. The fresh smell of sun-dried sheets is the relative absence of fungi in the desert created by putting the sheets in the sunshine. This is why the weather influences us so much. Cold and damp climates might not technically be making you ill, but when you consider how connected microbiota is to the weather, they might as well be. These shifts in weather allow microbes to proliferate and spread. Similarly, inside the body, a shift in heat, moisture and gases can cause certain microbiota to spread into regions which are not beneficial. This makes gas exchange a very important aspect of your climate barrier. As you inhale, microbiota come in; as you exhale, microbiota from your gut can rise into your mouth and spread to the outer landscape. They can go anywhere the gases allow them.

The life within you will thrive or die based on the kinds of gases that are available. Different mixtures of gases harbor their own particular forms of life. Some microbiota love nitrogen or hydrogen. Some prefer oxygen, while others can't stand it. They require the right degree of gases in order to thrive. As the ratio of gases shifts, some microbiota die and others begin to flourish. The balance of life is determined by the balance of gases.

GASOTRANSMITTERS

Gasotransmitters were discovered in the early 1990s and their discovery is redefining the way we think about medicine. They are small molecules of gas such as nitric oxide, hydrogen sulfide and carbon monoxide. They can pass freely through membranes and transmit signals from neurons to target cells.

Gasotransmitters are involved with nearly every process in the body. They have well-defined functions. Some send messages to tell cells how much energy they should be producing. When the right proportion of gasotransmitters pain stops and energy production goes up.

Chinese medicine has long recognized that gases within the body play a role in the warming, holding, and energizing of the human body, as well as providing communication throughout your systems. Medically there are names for many kinds of gases based on their actions in the body. While early Chinese medicine practitioners lacked the technology to identify and measure the exact gases, they were keenly aware of how these gases permeated the body and the points at which they exited the skin.

"Qi" (氣) literally means gas in Chinese. The pictograph shows steam 气 coming off of rice 米. A more ancient pictograph shows smoke coming off of fire. In either case, it refers to gases or vapors. This is a fundamental part of how yoga, acupuncture and meditation practices work.

COMPARISON OF QI AND GASOTRANSMITTERS

CHINESE MEDICINE'S CONCEPT OF QI "GAS"	GASOTRANSMITTERS
Can travel through the body	Can travel through the body
Provides a communication function in the body	Provides a communication function in the body
Is created by combining breath and food	A combination of gases drawn in from the lungs, amino acids and endogenous production from microbiota. Some gases such as nitric oxide can be synthesized from most cell types
Is influenced by a special gas in the kidneys, which is associated with sexual function	Hydrogen sulfide is a gasotransmitter associated with sexual function. It influences nitric oxide
Serves as a source of energy	Mitochondria release nitric oxide, which signals the breakdown of fat into usable energy and tell mitochondria to begin producing more ATP. ATP is the body's energy currency
When qi is unevenly distributed, it causes a lack of energy	Nitric oxide regulates metabolism of energy However, high concentrations of nitric oxide inhibit the mitochondrial respiration and limit energy production
Has a warming function	Nitric oxide converts fat into heat. It can improve the thermogenesis of brown fat
Is involved with the body's metabolism	Is involved with the body's metabolism

CHINESE MEDICINE'S CONCEPT OF QI "GAS"	GASOTRANSMITTERS
Has overlapping functions with nerves, but cannot be limited to nerves alone	Nerves release gasotransmitters which travel through membranes and make their way to other nerves. In the central and peripheral nervous system, nitric oxide serves as a neurotransmitter. In the nervous system, nitric oxide regulates neurotransmitter release and it can play a key role in synaptic plasticity and morphogenesis
Controls blood circulation and has a close relationship with blood	Nitric oxide dilates blood vessels, influencing blood circulation
Travels along acupuncture channels and exits at acupuncture points	Nitric oxide contents and neuronal nitric oxide synthase expression are consistently higher in the skin acupoints/meridians. Enhanced nitric oxide in the acupoints/meridians is generated from multiple resources
Too much causes inflammation. This is known as "liver qi stagnation"	Large amounts of nitric oxide, generated primarily by iNOS, can be toxic and cause inflammation, particularly oxidative damage to the liver
Influences water metabolism	Nitric oxide plays an important role in controlling enzymes such as sodium potassium ATPase. This enzyme is essential for the body's cellular pumps to control how much water is kept inside cells
Can be directed by intention	Neurotransmitters connect the brain and spinal cord with cells and peripheral neurons. These neurotransmitters release nitric oxide

CHINESE MEDICINE'S CONCEPT OF QI "GAS"	GASOTRANSMITTERS
Facilitates the actions of the internal organs and endocrine system	Facilitates the actions of the internal organs and endocrine system
Its even flow influences emotional states and endocrine function	Herbal formulas which have a sedative influence on the body seem to lower levels of nitric oxide. In addition, acupuncture therapy, which is used to regulate the flow of nitric oxide in the body, has been shown to be effective for depression
Controls gut balance	Nitric oxide kills off certain microorganisms while allowing others to thrive

NITRIC OXIDE AND INTESTINAL WAVES

The distribution of nitric oxide plays a major role in the rate at which food travels through your gastrointestinal system. It influences the wavelike movements in the intestines. If these waves move food slowly, the decay stays in the body and causes heat retention. If they move food through quickly, it causes heat loss as the feces leave your body. This is one method of temperature regulation in the body.

NITRIC OXIDE AND INSULIN FUNCTION

Nitric oxide stimulates pancreatic enzymes and hormones such as insulin. This helps you to utilize sugars efficiently. It also helps you to feel energetic and alert.

NITRIC OXIDE AND BLOOD CIRCULATION

Nitric oxide is involved in the regulation of regional blood flow. It dilates blood vessels and increases blood circulation. This increased blood flow helps every organ you can think of, from your brain to your kidneys. Nitric oxide is the basis for many popular pharmaceuticals such as Inomax and Viagra, which help increase blood flow to vital parts of the body. Nitric oxide can help you maintain a healthy heart and a healthy sex life[7].

NITRIC OXIDE AND FLEXIBILITY

One of the reasons that yoga, daoyin, qigong and martial arts put such an emphasis on the flow of gases through the

---

[7] *In an animal study on rats, nitric oxide effects on erectile dysfunction were demonstrated to be testosterone dependent. "Nitric oxide mediated erectile activity is a testosterone dependent event: a rat erection model." by Zvara P1, Sioufi R, Schipper HM, Begin LR, Brock GB.*

body is that it has a direct influence on relaxing smooth muscle, fascia, and tendons. Some people hold stretches with minimal gain. Isolating a muscle group may not be as good as relieving tension and improving the flow of nitric oxide throughout the body[8].

NITRIC OXIDE AND WATER METABOLISM

When people carry too much water in the cells, their metabolism becomes waterlogged and slows down. It can make them feel sluggish. This is because they can't distribute their energy efficiently. Imagine a flooded city. Transportation slows to a crawl. If you have fresh fruit, it won't be getting to grocery stores and will rot in the field while other people go hungry. The human body works in a similar fashion. When water metabolism breaks down, it hurts the body at a systemic level. Heavier people tend to have lower levels of sodium potassium ATPase than thin people. As a result, the heavier you get, the more likely it is that you are bogged down in water.

---

[8] *The other major inhibitor of flexibility is poor muscle balance. A lengthy subject unto itself.*

Sodium potassium ATPase helps your body's pumps to move water in and out of cells. Just as pumps keep water from flooding a city's subway systems, these sodium potassium pumps keep water from getting into places that should be dry. This water tends to drain downward, causing fungal infections in the lower parts of the body. This typically results in fungal infections of the toenails, yeast infections, jock itch or rashes and pimples on the insides of the legs. When this damp and wet environment stays for too long, the body begins to get swampy and slimy.

BIOFILMS

When your body holds the wrong kinds of gases, rapscallion microbes flourish. They grow resistant to antibiotics and learn to outsmart your immune system. When your body turns up the heat to cook them, they protect themselves by creating slimy dwellings called biofilms. These mucoid plaques are caused when your immune system tries to kill off bacteria through inflammation. They respond by creating a slimy protective environment to hide in until the attack blows over. They lie in wait until you get tired. When the coast is clear, they spread throughout your body. They begin slowly breaking you down. Biofilms are associated with a wide range of chronic diseases such as Parkinson's, diabetes, sleep apnea, inflammatory bowel disorders, colon cancer, and obesity.

One way to help dissolve them is to provide the body with a healthy flow of gasotransmitters. An unhealthy distribution of nitric oxide is associated with biofilms and obesity and sleep apnea. Thankfully, there are entire treatment modalities geared specifically to adjust the flow of gasotransmitters in the body.

GASOTRANSMITTERS AND ACUPUNCTURE

By measuring for lower electrical resistance, Dr. Jia-Xu Chen and Sheng-Xing Ma were able to find the exact positions of acupuncture points. They discovered nitric oxide at levels 2–3 times higher on acupuncture points than at other places on the skin's surface. Acupuncturists work directly with gasotransmitters, which pass through membranes, communicate with other nerves and act directly on cells. It tells them to start producing energy and turn fat into heat. By controlling the flow of nitric oxide, acupuncturists can influence the body's rate of metabolism and reduce inflammation. They use needling techniques to control the flow of energy production by releasing this gas at strategic exits, similar to exits on a freeway.

If you have a traffic jam, you have a lot of power available in those cars. Each car can go faster than 100 miles per hour and pull a great deal of weight. Unfortunately, within the context of a traffic jam, each car might as well be a donkey because the cars can't travel at their optimum speed. The problem isn't a lack of energy; it's a problem of distribution. The key to unlocking all that power is to reduce the number of cars on the road. This optimizes the number of cars that can work efficiently for transportation. In the same way, your body requires an even flow of gasotransmitters in order to do its best work. Inserting a needle creates an "off ramp" for the extra gasotransmitters to escape and improve the ergonomics of its flow.

HYDROGEN SULFIDE

The ancient Chinese believed there was a gas in the kidneys (kidney qi) that was associated with a grouping of diseases such as kidney failure, obesity, short lifespan, poor sexual function, poor memory, disrupted sleep cycles, high blood pressure, elevated fear response, and temperature regulation.

COMPARISON OF KIDNEY QI AND HYDROGEN SULFIDE

CHINESE MEDICINE'S CONCEPT OF KIDNEY QI	HYDROGEN SULFIDE
Associated with water, often called, "source gas"	Feeds bacteria in hydrothermal vents, which use it as an energy source in the depths of the ocean. Very likely the source of life on this planet
Declines with age	Declines with age
Influences longevity	In animal studies hydrogen sulfide has shown the ability to extend lifespan by switching on a gene called *Klotho*
Related to sexual function	Related to sexual function
Affects hormones	Affects hormones
Affects blood pressure	Affects blood pressure
Regulates temperature	Regulates temperature
Related to kidney disease, obesity and diabetes	Related to kidney disease, obesity and type 2 diabetes

CARBON MONOXIDE

Carbon monoxide regulates cell death, thins blood and is influential in where new blood vessels form. It also serves an important role in cerebrovascular circulation.

MEDITATION AND GASOTRANSMITTERS

Taiji and Zen meditation have been shown to increase gasotransmitters while decreasing oxidation.

QIGONG

Qigong is the practice of regulating gasotransmitters. This helps to regulate inflammation, reduce stress, and increase the efficiency of energy balance in the body. The range of qigong techniques is quite diverse. Some exercises are done lying down, while others are highly athletic. Qigong exercises and therapies have been shown to be effective in the treatment and management of fibromyalgia.

YOGA

Yoga is an Indian philosophical school of thought. The postures or "asanas" typically associated with yoga have specific health effects on the body. Practicing these asanas has been shown to be helpful for people with fibromyalgia.

AEROBICS

Aerobic activity is beneficial for increased blood circulation and gas exchange in the body. Aerobic exercise, like qigong, has been shown to have beneficial effects on fibromyalgia.

TAI CHI

Tai chi or "taijiquan" is a martial art typically practiced in a slow and meditative way. It combines breath and movement to become a form of active qigong. It is particularly renowned for helping with balance, regulating blood sugar, and helping with chronic pain and depression. It has been shown to be very effective for fibromyalgia pain.

CHINESE MEDICINE

Chinese medicine as a whole is beneficial for tender points. Because all acupuncture will improve the overall flow of nitric oxide. There are acupuncture methods that can be effective in the treatment of fibromyalgia.

EXERCISE: STOMACH MASSAGE

Stomach massage is an incredibly efficient exercise for alleviating gut dysbiosis[9].

1. Fold your hands so that the webs of your hands are pressed

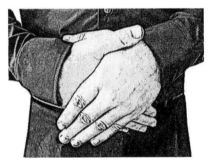

together.

2. Take a deep breath so that your abdomen pushes outward. Abdominal breathing is a crucial and often overlooked part of digestion.

3. Straighten your posture.

4. Press your joined hand against your abdomen. Create intra-abdominal pressure using your diaphragm and

the pressure from your hands pushing inward.

5. Begin massaging your abdomen in a counter clockwise direction 36 times.

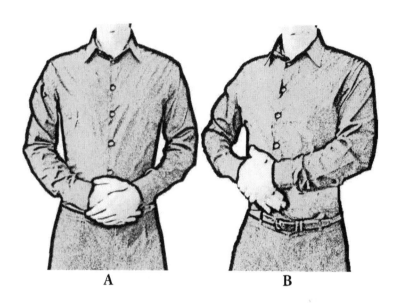

A   **B**

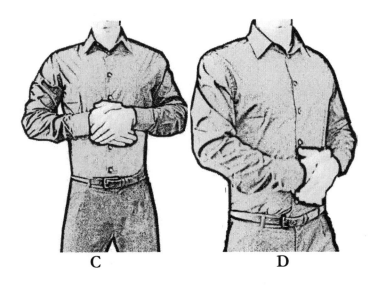

C   D

6. Reverse direction and continue to massage 36 times in circles.

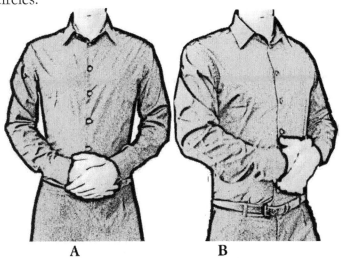

A   B

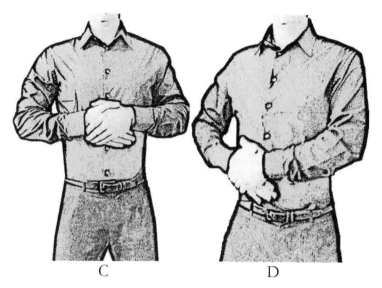

C	D

7. Once you begin to belch or pass wind, you can lighten the pressure on your arms. Continue massaging and start using your whole body, following the motion of your hands. Don't worry about doing it perfectly; just get the methane out.

8. When you are finished, bring your hands to your lower abdomen and breathe gently using your diaphragm for 8 breaths.

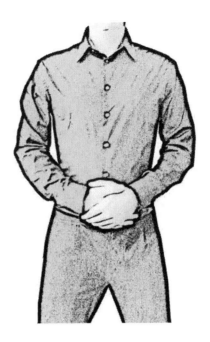

Chapter 15: Emotional Factors

"Eating is so intimate. It's very sensual. When you invite someone to sit at your table and you want to cook for them, you're inviting a person into your life."

—*Maya Angelou*

FIBROMYALGIA AND PSYCHOLOGY

A Cochrane review of medical literature found that the effects of psychological treatments for fibromyalgia are comparable to those reported for other pain and drug treatments. Cognitive-behavioral therapy was found to be associated with the largest effect sizes.

PSYCHOLOGICAL FACTORS: GEARING DOWN AND GETTING TO SLEEP

Change can cause tension. This is a natural response that helps people stay alert and adapt. The stress comes; it makes you alert; you deal with the challenge and move on. Over time, tension can build up. Stress in life is like wind on a tree: its effects are often unnoticed. The branches bend and circle back. If the tree never gets sufficient relief from the wind, it becomes windswept. Long-term stress leaves a lasting impression. This impression often manifests as fat gain, poor flexibility, and lower energy levels. Ultimately this can all be attributed to poor sleep.

Most of our body's repair happens while we are sleeping. It's the time you are losing fat, adjusting psychologically and getting stronger.

Stress hormones like cortisol act as our alarm clock. They signal you to wake up in the morning. If they are too prevalent, they can keep you alert when you really don't need to be. From sleepovers as a kid I learned not to be the first one to fall asleep. I learned through my socialization that falling asleep was rude and a sign of laziness. Besides that, it left you vulnerable to attack or having someone play a prank on you. Like many Americans, I thought this life was normal until I discovered that the fear of sleeping was pretty bizarre.

My friend Biagio is from a family that never allowed people to play pranks on sleeping people. As a result, they can put their heads down and sleep in any position. Once asleep, you can crank up the music and nothing seems to stir them. I wondered how this was possible and he explained it like this: "There are many social taboos in society against sleeping. People will say you are lazy or it is seen as rude, but for some reason it's perfectly acceptable to watch hours of television per day. The next time you have nothing to do, just tell yourself it's okay to sleep."

While he was saying this, his father Jaime came in and weighed in on the topic. "Many people are afraid to sleep because they think some bad guys will come and kill them, but no one is going to get you. The whole idea is just insane.

Actually, sleeping in public makes the environment more relaxed and allows other people to relax, too. Sure, maybe someone will steal your wallet, but in my whole life, no one has and if they did it, they would steal less money than it costs for a visit to see a psychologist. I feel so relaxed that I don't need to take vacations to unwind. If you need to escape your life to feel healthy and happy, there is a big problem."

These weren't the naively optimistic words of someone who had led a sheltered life. Jaime was a child soldier in the Bolivian wars that eventually lead to independence in 1952. He took his first bullet when he was six. Three days before his seventh birthday, a Spanish sniper was killing civilians in a market. Jamie used his small size to flank him and put a bullet through his skull. After Bolivia gained independence, the UN and Peace Corps helped place Jaime in a foster home in the U.S. By the time he was in middle school, he had seen more stress, violence, and hardship than most Americans see in their entire lifetimes. He followed a path from violence to inner tranquility that was passed down from his ancestors.

WISDOM OF TEARS

One of the most important lessons I learned from Jaime was to cry. When we cry, we release stress hormones through our tears. He explained that we should think of it like urination. Not urinating for 20 years doesn't make you strong – it makes you broken. Jaime's ancestors, the Inca, worshiped the sun and paid special attention to it. They considered the sun to be akin to the human heart. When the sky is dark and overcast, the sun is hidden. As the rain falls, the clouds disperse and the sun shines brightly through the darkness. When we are sad, our heart becomes blocked by clouds of despair. As our tears fall like rain, the sadness parts and our hearts shine through. This cycle of joy and sadness is just part of the human experience. It is the same as the cycles of rain and sunshine which keep a forest healthy.

THE POWER OF SILENCE

Few things are as healing as spending time in the woods. Losing yourself in nature's rhythms is one of the best ways to restore yourself.

Lt. Troy Givens had his legs blown apart by an improvised explosive device while stationed in Afghanistan. As a hunter he understood the power of being quiet in nature as a way to restore himself. When he returned home, he went camping. Now, Troy takes vets who have a high level of post-traumatic stress into the woods for a week. He explains that "by day five, they are good".

There is a time when it's best to simply get out of your head and into a steady rhythm. This is a good way to attune to nature's principles and restore your innate harmony.

EMOTIONAL FACTORS

There are strong links between poor psychological health, particularly from bad childhood experiences, and obesity. This increased stress response can contribute to fat gain. Adverse reactions from childhood can cause behavioral disorders as people sabotage their efforts to heal due to conditioning they received along the way. If they identify with abuse or neglect, they may feel as though they are unworthy of proper care. This contributes to many people "letting themselves go" and not taking proper care of their bodies.

To improve your state of self-care it's important to identify and reverse negative conditioning. This starts with identifying the voices you may have recorded and replay to yourself. To varying degrees, people hold themselves to the level of their expectations and frame their worldview based on language. Someone might curse you once, but if you play that in your head on a continual loop, the curse can become a repeating pattern in your life.

Dr. Scott Pengelly is a clinical health psychologist who works in behavioral medicine. He has helped many people, from those with morbid obesity to high-level athletes. He teaches his patients to look for verbal cues that will either cue them for success or curse them for failure. He calls these verbal cues "canaries in a coalmine" and explains it like this: "In the past, miners kept canaries with them as they traveled into the bowels of the earth. When the canary died, they knew they were in danger of gas poisoning. In the same way, these verbal cues will help you to discover something about your mental programming."

EXERCISE: CHANGE THE TAPE

Pay attention to how you speak to yourself. If the words you tell yourself are negative, change your internal recording. This is no easy task, and it takes time. Pay attention to the types of words you use in your daily life. Begin to notice how these words impact your expectations and self-image. Adjust your internal and external vocabulary so that it is in line with your desired outcome.

STRESS, DIGESTION AND BLOOD CIRCULATION

Your blood does not flow evenly to all parts of the body at the same time. It couldn't. It needs an area that is relatively empty to allow for flow. When you are hot, blood travels to the exterior to allow excess heat to radiate through the skin to the outside world. When we are cold, the opposite happens. Blood circulation will change its relative position during periods of activity and rest. It will alter slightly based on the time of day and the time of year. This is largely regulated by hormones. Someone may feel "cold feet" on their wedding day because the stress response is causing the body to hold blood near the organs for protection. Too much stress can interfere with the healthy distribution of blood and hormones.

EXERCISE: FEEL THE PULSE[9]

Feel how your blood is flowing with every beat of your heart. Feel its waves travel through your body. If you feel an obstruction, relax and imagine the blood flowing through to the tips of your toes and fingers. If you can feel your blood reaching the branches of your body, then you have good circulation. If not, then take care of this right now. Lie down and feel your heart beating. Follow the blood and feel for the waves. By looking internally, your entire body becomes an MRI. You can see where there are obstructions and feel whether your blood is more to the interior or exterior of the body.

TEMPERAMENT

When you alter your gut and gasotransmitters, you can

---

[9] *Credit to Mathew Lowes*

adapt your emotional state and personality. The word "temperament" shares a common root with the words "temper" and "temperature". It comes from the idea that the climate of the human body affects personality. This idea is found throughout the world in various plant-based medical systems.

The common thread of these traditions is using the internal "temperature" to influence emotional states. This is something science is rediscovering. The gut and gasotransmitters influence the brain in ways we are just beginning to understand. Mental illnesses are becoming increasingly associated with changes in gut microbiota. Nitric oxide is directly involved in the neurobiology of major depression. If you want to change your temperament, begin with your internal climate.

Chapter 16: The Light Within

"Your body is woven from the light of heaven."

—*Rumi*

ELECTRICITY, GAS AND LIGHT

Your brain is composed of billions of specialized cells called neurons. They transfer information throughout your nervous system. This is how messages are transferred from electricity to chemicals and back again. Neurons communicate in several ways. While you are probably familiar with the electrical connection, they also release gases, sound waves and frequencies of light. Gases and light both serve to increase communication in the body[10].

The frequency of your brainwaves causes your nerves to fire at different rates, illuminating the darkest parts of our body like lighting shooting across the night sky.

Within your cells' nucleus, light is constantly being

---

[10] *It's entirely possible that sound also acts as a carrier of information. I just haven't found any solid research one way or the other.*

absorbed and emitted by DNA molecules. The biophotons emissions change, leaving a signature of light as unique as your fingerprint. This signature changes depending on its state of health. When cells are injured or cancerous, they change their light pattern. Cells appear to use this light as an intricate system of communication. This is how they complain to their neighbor or ask to borrow tools they never intend to return. It is also how they call for an ambulance when they are injured. When cells are damaged they release a different light signature, which attracts stem cells to be delivered through the tiny tubes called Bonghan ducts.

You can also influence how much light they emit by thinking. Research has demonstrated that simply imagining light or setting your mind to different brainwave patterns can alter the rate of biophoton emissions. By learning to control your brainwave frequency, you may be influencing cellular communication.

BRAINWAVES – THE RHYTHM OF LIGHT

Because thinking kicks up such a bioelectric storm, it's possible to measure the skin to see changes in electrical activity. It is easy to tell if you are thinking, sleeping, or dreaming by looking at the patterns made by the electroencephalogram (EEG) machine. This demonstrates that your thoughts have a powerful influence on your entire system. Changes in your brainwave patterns can influence your emotions and how your digestive system works. This directly affects your microbial garden.

There is no ideal brainwave state. You need to flexibly change depending on your needs. Getting stuck in any one of them is a sign of a problem. Being in a state of spiritual ecstasy is great, but if you can't integrate that into your life and come back down to Earth, then it's a sign of mental illness. On the other hand, constantly being asleep means that you are in a coma. Having the ability to shift between mental states is a better sign of health.

Being able to smoothly transfer between mental states is important for your health, both mentally and physically. There is a time to be at a high frequency and a time to be at a low frequency. These follow each other just like seasonal and daily cycles. The transfer between the low and high frequency brainwaves is just another wave. The smoother the wave, the better the flow of energy.

Gamma waves are associated with prayer, meditation and language learning in small children. At 40 pulses per second, this is the brain sprinting.

When we you alert or agitated, our brainwave setting is typically on "beta" and it ranges from 13–60 pulses per second. This is where many people set themselves. If you get stuck in this frequency, you tend to waste energy on worry and it can result in having a racing mind that can interfere with sleep.

In alpha waves, your brainwaves slow to a more manageable 7–13 pulses per second. This relaxed focus allows us to feel mentally clear and makes it easier to remember information. It is also the frequency most associated with biophoton light.

When you are relaxed and getting sleepy, you are in theta brainwaves. Your brain pulses between 4–7 beats per second. It is associated with memory, sensory awareness, movement, automatic walking and other activities governed by your hippocampus.

When your brain waves are around 0.1–4 pulses per

second, you are in delta. This is a deep state of sleep.

COST IN ENERGY

Your brain uses between 20–30 percent of your body's energy. That makes your thoughts pretty expensive. The brain will also take what it needs. Using it too much can cause food cravings which serve your brain more than the rest of your body. When the brain demands sugar faster than the body can supply it, it causes a sweet tooth, making you crave sugars to satiate the craving as quickly as possible. While this is great for your brain, your digestive system can get bogged down. The influx of sugars makes the body get less efficient and it creates a downward spiral. This imbalance is caused by thinking more than moving. It is what happens when you focus too much on the outside world and lose touch with your instincts.

INTUITIVE AND LOGICAL

You have the ability to think both logically and intuitively. Intuitive thinking is based on how you interact with your natural instincts. Unless you take time to think, it is unlikely that you will come to any sort of logical conclusion. You also need to take time to get in touch with your instincts and subconscious mind to help preserve yourself. Your subconscious mind is made of everything you see, hear and experience. You can't focus on all of it, so most of it gets stored. Think of it like all of the frequencies on a radio. If you were to hear them all at once, it would sound like gibberish and noise. By tuning in to one, you get clear reception, but are deaf to what happens on the other radio stations.

In a study on intentional blindness, people were asked to watch a video of two basketball teams, one wearing white and the other wearing black. Both groups were mixed into a relatively small space and each group passed a basketball among their teammates. Both groups moved about randomly. Participants in the study were asked to count the number of passes the white team performed. As this was happening, a man in a gorilla suit walked among the players, stood there for a second and then walked off-screen. In most groups 50 percent of the people were so focused on the passes that they failed to notice the gorilla. When you get too caught up in one way of viewing the world, it can blind you to other vantage points.

To get a full perspective, change the dial on your brainwaves. You can tune into the different frequencies of your own consciousness. Some of these frequencies carry valuable information about your body. Your instincts may be telling you vital information about your body's inner workings. They are walking through like the gorilla in the experiment, but if you are focused only on one vantage point, you won't get the message. Tapping into the other aspects of your perception is a source of tremendous power. Many great thinkers have found inspiration while dreaming or in a state of prayer. Einstein used daydreaming as a way to spark creativity. Your instincts are just beyond the borders of your rational mind. They are there waiting for you to access them. All you have to do it tap in. A great way to do this is to learn from your breathing.

SIGHING

When people are stressed, they naturally sigh. This is how the body blows off steam and relaxes. The exhalation of the sigh is more forceful than the inhalation. How do people breathe when they are hot or stressed? They exhale forcefully with a "hhhaaaa" sound. It is similar to the way a dog pants on a hot day. How do people breathe when they are angry? They tend to shout, forcing out air with every breath. It relates to how people swear when they are stressed or use Lamaze breathing during childbirth to alleviate pain – it's quite literally how we vent. It's how we expel. It's how we cough. Learn from this.

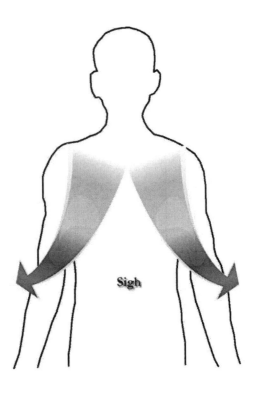

Sigh

YAWNING

When you yawn, you take a huge breath in and then seem to hold it. This is a powerful lesson we would do well to learn from.

Think of what happens when you are taking a shower and the water suddenly goes cold. You immediately gasp by inhaling into your chest. This is a yawn. From this, you can discover how to warm and strengthen the body. If you find yourself yawning during the day, exaggerate your breathing pattern in order to recharge. When we feel cold and sad, you use a similar style of breathing to literally inspire ourselves. You have heard of people being inspired or venting. This knowledge is part of the human experience and its traces have been left in our language. If you need to chill out, then sigh. If you need to power up, then yawn. At the root, breathing exercises boil down to this.

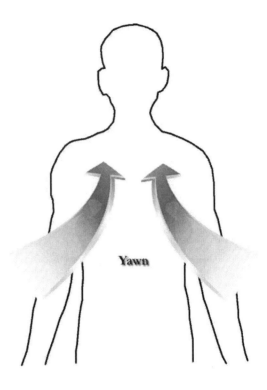

MASTERING YOUR MIND WITH BREATHING

Your emotions and breathing patterns affect each other. When you are in a state of fear, your breathing will be high in the chest; when you're in a state of peace, your breathing will cause your abdomen to expand the way a baby breathes at rest.

In the animal kingdom, predators are keenly attuned to breathing and movement. The freeze response limits moving and breathing to help animals hide. This can stifle your breathing during times of stress. Aside from freezing, there is a fight-or-flight response. This can set breathing higher in the chest compared to the lower abdominal breathing you might see when an infant is sleeping. Your emotional state will change your breathing pattern. The flip side to this is that you can alter your breathing patterns to either excite yourself or make yourself more active. They work in feedback loops that are at once automatic and also under your control. Sometimes it can be difficult to accurately gauge your emotional state. A good system check for the human body is to learn from your breathing patterns.

EXERCISE: LISTENING TO YOUR BREATHING

Observe your breath and see what you can learn about yourself. Simply observe the waves of breath the way you might watch waves on the beach. Observe it without trying to control it. Simply allow it to work by itself. Try to see how deeply you are breathing.

-Is your breath making a sound?

-Is it easier to inhale or exhale?

-How does the way you are breathing influence your pain?

-Which parts of your body could use more ventilation?

-Do your cells want more or less oxygen?

-Are you "yawning" by drawing in more air and holding it, or "sighing" by exhaling with more force?

-Are there any areas of tension that are inhibiting your breathing?

-How do different emotional states influence your breathing?

FASTING

Fasting is willingly abstaining from food for a period of time. It is a cultural and religious practice found throughout the world. People fast for social, spiritual and health purposes. Many people who fast describe feelings of alertness, mood improvements and sometimes euphoria.

Fasting affects blood sugar and brainwave patterns. This is why people are told not to eat before getting an EEG to scan their brainwaves – it helps the test to be accurate. Fasting can increase insulin sensitivity, and lower cholesterol and blood pressure.

There are many proponents who tout the benefits of fasting. Like anything else, it depends on context. Fasting can make you feel cold, weak and cranky as your microbiota influences your opioid receptors and start screaming for attention. This can drive up cortisol levels that are associated with stress and pain signaling. On top of this, blood-sugar drops make people grumpy. If your body isn't ready, then fasting will only serve to drive up pain signals.

From a traditional Chinese medical perspective, fasting serves to dry and cool the body. If your body is too warm and moist, this may be a beneficial practice. Fasting has its benefits, but you should make sure you have a strong foundation before you begin.

If your body is working efficiently, then skipping a few meals won't bother you. If your body is already regulated, it starts using your glycogen and fat supplies for energy. It will diminish the hunger mechanism and you will have less opioid noise from microbiota. Then you can enjoy the benefits of fasting while limiting the side effects.

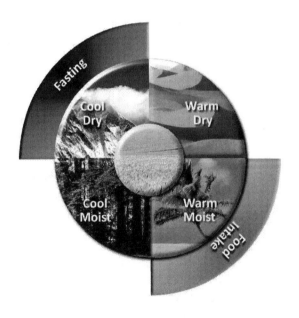

HORMONE BALANCE

Hormonal fluctuations influence fat storage. As people age, there is a decline in sex hormones. These decline faster with stress. With hormonal imbalance, diet and exercise stop being as effective for maintaining energy balance. If you suspect that hormone imbalance is impeding your health, a good strategy is to get a hormone panel and see a doctor.

DRINK THE SUN

When you get proper amounts of sunlight, it triggers melanocortins, peptide hormones that have biphasic actions on pain signals. Sunlight is vital for regulating circadian rhythms. The optic nerve in your eye receives important light signals that set your biological clock to help you maintain hormonal alignment with the heavens. Sleeping at night will allow you to get normal spikes in melatonin, which helps to regulate fat storage and pain signaling. Your natural amount of melatonin will vary throughout the year, affecting behavior and pain levels. In the winter you are supposed to sleep more, while in the summer, you can enjoy more of the evenings. This is the effect of the seasons on all living things. Your body wants to adapt, and you would be wise to let it do its job.

Artificial light can mess with these ingrained signals, but there are ways around it. First is the understanding that just because you have lights doesn't mean you must turn them on. The second is that you can get blue light-filtering glasses to remind your body to start producing melatonin. Start to wear them at sunset. This can help you get to sleep earlier and regulate your natural hormonal cycles.

. KNOW THYSELF

EXERCISE: SYSTEMS CHECK PART 1

Before a plane takes off, the crew does a systems check to ensure that everything is working properly. Even if they fly the plane every day and are fairly certain everything is in good order, they check again because it's really important that the airplane doesn't crash and make paraplegics out of the few survivors. This is particularly important with older planes. The mechanics can replace parts, but as the plane gets older it becomes increasingly prone to breaking down. Your body also is constantly making repairs, but over time it becomes more prone to breaking down. Systematic checking of the body's systems is a wise thing to do, especially since you only get one body in this life[11].

1. Begin by lying down and relaxing. Visualize the top of your head and scan slowly downward towards your feet. If you feel tension, then relax it and move on.

2. Once you reach your feet, do the reverse, imagining the insides of your feet and visualizing the body up toward the crown of your head.

3. Next, visualize your body going from the outside layers to the inside, going as deep as your bone marrow. Take mental notes of any areas of pain or tension.

4. Finally, go from the deepest part of your body to the outside.

EXERCISE: SYSTEMS CHECK PART 2

This type of self-evaluation happens throughout the day

---

[11] *Credit to Matt Lowes*

and is made up of five questions.[12]

1. How are your liquids? Do you need more or less water? Is your urine yellow or clear?

2. How is your emotional state? How are you adapting to your external circumstances? Are you in an emotional state that is not relevant to your present moment?

3. How is your circulatory system? Do you bruise easily? Do your hands or feet feel cold? Do you have chronic pain?

4. How is your internal microbiome? What does your tongue look like? How is your appetite? What are your bowel movements like? Do you have lots of gas? Are you bloated after meals?

5. How is your respiration? Can you easily take deep breaths? Do you easily feel winded during exercise?

EXERCISE: FEEL YOUR FOOD

---

[12] *Credit to James Shyun OMD Ph.D*

To get a better understanding of your internal satiation, feel food when you swallow it. Feel it all the way through your body. You have a nervous system dedicated to it. If you pay attention to what you are doing, you might just do a better job. More often than not, people don't give themselves the proper time to eat, break down, and assimilate their nutrition. When you take the time to do this, you paradoxically create more usable time. When you are healthy and more energetic, you will need less time to rest and can use that time to accomplish all of your daily tasks. You can make this a meditation exercise. Close your eyes and feel your food. Ask yourself an hour later where it is. With a little practice, you will be able to increase your ability to detect what is going on. This alone is one of the most powerful tools for weight loss, energy accumulation, and peace of mind.[13]

---

[13] *Credit to Jaime Arobba*

Part III

Chapter 17: Mastering Movement

"People are born supple and soft. When dead they are stiff and hard. Plants are born tender and pliant, at death they are brittle and dry. Whoever is stiff and inflexible is a student of death. Whoever is soft and yielding is a student of life. The hard and stiff will be broken. The soft and supple will endure."

—*Laozi*

UNDERSTANDING MOVEMENT

Where there is life, there are rhythms and waves. There is a pulsatile wave as blood moves through your body. There is rhythm to the waves of your cerebrospinal fluid, which are bathing your brain and allowing you to read these words. Your brain moves and is shaped with every beat of your heart. Your cells have a rhythmic plasticity. By waves, you swallow food. By waves, the food travels through your intestines. You are now breathing in cycles of steady and rhythmic breaths and the vibrations in your larynx give you a voice. Maintaining the flow of the forces in your body is the key to moving well.

Your body is constantly suffering shock. That's a good thing. It's an important part of life and these forces can help you. By using relaxation and breathing, you can smooth out the edges caused by life's changes. It's the difference from being brushed by someone passing you on a busy street and slamming directly into them. By keeping your body loose, you allow the forces that travel through you with every step to slide off of you, rather than stopping in your joints and internal organs.

Having relaxed and even breathing allows you to move smoothly. It gives you additional circles to round out the forces that are constantly spiraling through your body. As you breathe, your whole body undulates and circles. If you hold your arm straight in front of you and breathe, you will notice that it rises and falls with your breath. As you study it further, you'll notice that the movement isn't linear, but elliptical. Breathing allows your motion to become smoother and helps you to find circles in every motion.

It can seem mysterious why a drunk person can sustain a vicious car crash with minimal injury while another person can trip and die. The difference is largely due to whether the forces move through the body or get trapped within. Falling down is really not a big deal. The fall only introduces force to the body. If the force goes around or through you, then it minimizes the amount of shock you absorb. What injures people is their own fear and tension. It locks forces inside the body. If instead of holding tension, you relax and smoothly exhale, it can help to reduce injury and make your landing smooth and round.

COMBINING BREATH AND MOVEMENT

The exploration of structure, movement and breathing is at the core of physical endeavors ranging from walking to triathlons. The best way to move well is to coordinate your actions with your breathing. If you push a heavy object, you naturally exhale with the force. You can apply this same principle to every motion.

If you are moving into alignment or drawing your hands and feet toward your center, then inhale. If you are extending outward or sitting down, then exhale softly and smoothly.

As an experiment, hold your breath and grab a glass of water, and bring it to your lips. Then repeat the same motion while exhaling as your hand extends toward the glass and inhaling as it comes in. You can inhale as you stand up and exhale as you sit down. Experiment with breathing and motion to find what is comfortable for you. You can make this moving meditation part of your daily life. With a hectic schedule and no time, you can still change your perspective and breathing to make use of the postures and movements that are already essential to your everyday routine. With every action you can relax and strengthen yourself.

As you move, you will find postures and activities which are less comfortable. If there is discomfort, there is undue tension. You then have two choices: You can either avoid the activity, or learn to use the postures to recognize and release undue tension[14]. If you are in the back seat of a small car or twisted in a yoga posture, the challenge is the same. It is learning to adjust your posture, breathing and mental state to make even uncomfortable situations pleasant. If you are averse to movement, learning to adapt in this way is the first step. By combining breath and movement you can begin to move with the fluidity and grace of a wild animal. If you need inspiration, then look at how oceanic animals swim, how birds fly and how running animals seem to ripple over the landscape. There is an effortless relaxation in even their most determined motions. This is what you can reclaim by

---

[14] *Bone spurs, tumors and shrapnel aside.*

combining breath and movement.

RELAXATION AND POSTURE

STANDING

Relaxation and breathing are the foundations of posture and movement. Many martial arts use standing posture holding and standing meditation as a way to perfect posture. They will stand in one place for up to an hour using as little muscular tension as possible to hold their posture. In the long run, this saves time and energy. By taking the time to release the emergency brakes in the body, it gives them the alignment to move quickly, issue power and sustain crushing blows without injury. Without relaxation and breathing, even daily activities become dangerous. Muscular tension pulls the body out of alignment. People often undergo surgery to align vertebrae that are only held out of alignment by their own muscular tension. In many cases, removing the tension is enough to allow the spine to find its natural alignment. Most people are stronger than they know – they are just living with tension. It's like driving around with the brakes on while your car is out of alignment. Before long you are out of gas and in need of expensive repairs.

SITTING

When you sit down, feel whether your posture is impeding your breathing, and use your breathing to open up and align your sitting position. As you inhale, straighten up; as you exhale, release excess tension. Use your breath to make your position as comfortable as possible.

USE EVERY MOMENT

If you are waiting in line somewhere, identify where your posture is off and use breathing to relax and align yourself. Remember this and you will never waste time again. Eventually we all get stuck somewhere. Perhaps it's a pointless meeting that carries on because some blowhard likes the sound of his own voice. Maybe it's a high-school graduation where you are subjected to a barrage of platitudes. We've all been there and you will probably have to attend more of these things in the future. Think of it as an intense yoga posture. Go inward, find your alignment and use breathing to make the situation useful. There is usually something that isn't flowing as well as it could. Relax your body, meditate with your eyes open, clap when you are supposed to and make the best of it. You can even smile, nod and give packaged responses without having to really be there mentally. In this way, you can make the experience restorative rather than soul-sucking.

If you don't want to meditate, you can just sleep. Lan and I used to be active with the Lions Club. Other than the two of us, most of the Lions in our chapter were well over 70 years old. Every Wednesday at lunch, different speakers came in. Some of them were great, but some had political agendas or were simply dull. When a speaker didn't connect with the audience, you would know it. A number of the members would simply go to sleep. Many weren't even subtle about it, with mouths agape and snoring. Some would even put their heads on the table. I thought there must be an epidemic of narcolepsy. As I investigated, I found that for some of them it was a conscious choice. I asked some of the members why they nodded off at times. One man answered, "Well, it beats getting upset over nothing." Another man was over 90 years old and active in the club. He gave me the following advice: "Imagine if all the idiots and the arguments were all just gone. You are better off getting some rest so that you have more energy for the things that actually matter." This may be sage advice, but unless you are retired, you might consider faking attention. After you retire, go ahead and sleep.

EXERCISE: LYING DOWN AND STANDING UP

One of the biggest dangers in life is falling down. This is a great exercise to get used to falling smoothly. When you go to bed, you can use your arms to robotically place yourself, or you can exhale smoothly and flow into a supine position. As your arm touches down, roll your forearm and relax with your breathing. If your breathing is fast, your movement should be fast. If you want to lie down gradually, then exhale slowly and allow your movement to follow your breathing. When you wake in the morning, you can begin to sit up as you inhale. Imagine that the air is pumping you upward. Falling down and bumping into things is part of life. With this daily exercise, you can discover how to minimize damage. With enough practice and training, it's possible for people to fall on pavement and rise again with ease. It can become so gentle that it is actually comfortable. Learning to fall is a skill martial artists use and one that everyone can benefit from.[15]

WALKING

While walking, continue to maintain relaxation and begin looking at how hard your heel strikes the ground. It is normal

---

[15] *Credit to Matt Lowes*

for the heel to touch first, but wait until your foot is flat on the ground to apply weight. Use calm and even breathing and look at how you can relax your legs to absorb shock. Make your movement poised and graceful. As you walk, begin to discover the figure-eight movement in your hips that occurs whenever you transfer weight from one foot to the other.

EXERCISE: LEARN FLUIDITY FROM WATER

Fill a bowl about halfway with water and place it on your head. I recommend using a plastic or metal bowl in case it falls off. As you walk, you can feel the changes in alignment by the way the water shifts in the bowl. This is a great exercise for improving your posture and ability to move well.[16]

ASCENDING STAIRS

While ascending stairs, focus more on the inhalation to get more oxygen into your system. Breathe like you are yawning. Draw your breath in using your abdomen, filling it up into your rib cage and passively allowing yourself to exhale.

---

[16] *Credit to James Shyun OMD. Ph.D*

DESCENDING STAIRS

While descending stairs, breathe more like you are sighing. This relaxes the hips and allows you to flow down the stairs. The inhalation provides a vertical cycle of motion, while relaxing the hips allows them to create a figure-eight motion. The combination of these three circles lets you make a vertical descent smoother. There are Daoists in Sichuan who use this method to flow down steep, slippery mountains that would cause other people to stumble and become injured. They travel quickly and smoothly. They seem to be floating more than running. This is called lightness skill and it has been exaggerated in literature and film to show people flying around on bamboo, running on water or jumping from one mountain to the next. In reality it's simply what happens when people free themselves of extra tension and begin to move with the grace and speed they were born to have.

In your daily life, you might not need to make a controlled fall down the side of a mountain, but you will probably encounter stairs. Stairs can be especially challenging for heavier people who have joint pain. By using these methods, you can make your descent as gentle as possible.[17]

DISCOVERING NATURAL ATHLETICISM

It can be challenging to keep up with a small child. For their size, they are surprisingly fast, with the kind of athleticism you find in most animals. Over time, most people love this natural athleticism. Kids follow the same gaits, breathing patterns and levels of tension modeled by adults. Eventually, the lessons they learn from observing adults can do more harm than good. To break these unhealthy patterns, you must begin training in alignment and relaxation to rediscover your natural poise. The softening exercises described here should take a higher priority with age until they become the majority of one's activities at the end of life.

If you observe a tiger or any wild animal, you can see how its whole body pumps its lungs. From the lower abdomen to the rib cage, the whole system undulates. This is an important part of digestion as it massages the internal organs, particularly the intestines. As your body becomes more in tune with your natural rhythms, your senses sharpen.

---

[17] *Credit to Kevin Loftus and Liu Sui Bing*

This increases your physical awareness of what you are eating and allows you to process it more effectively. This approach to movement is about remembering what you once knew and letting go of the things that have come to stand in your way. You can forget copying the disjointed movements of others and remember how fast you ran for your size as a kid. Think of how you ran barefoot over rocks and up into trees.

MOVING WITH JOY

Consider how children misbehave in grocery stores. If they are angry, they tend to stay in one place, kicking and screaming and flailing about. When they are happy and playing, they can run several laps around a grocery store. At some level we are all still little kids. When we are stressed, we don't move very much and act like jerks. The message boards of the Internet demonstrate that there are plenty of people who don't feel like moving, but do feel like throwing a tantrum and insulting anyone who comes near them. All of this is just a grown-up version of flailing about and screaming in the grocery store. It's better to be the kid running around and laughing. If you are playing, you feel like moving. When kids are sitting for hours on end and the recess bell finally rings, they run out the door. Dogs do the same thing. When you reach a point where you can sit down for hours and don't want to get out and move, you are sick. If you aren't bursting with energy and find it normal to sit down all day and then go home to sit and watch television, you have nothing in common with a wild animal. This means that your energy levels are too low. Look for a feeling of life and movement in your muscles. If you feel this, then you are on the right track.

SOFT LEGS

Many people walk as though they are on stilts. It's as if their legs are two columns that they rock back and forth on. Using this method of walking puts incredible stress on the knees, hips and lower back; it's a poor way to move. Even a crane with its long slender legs will bend them with delicacy, precision and softness. Wild animals do not clamber. They don't throw one leg in front of the other and fall onto it. On uneven terrain, this is an easy way to get injured. The world of ice and moss and sharp rocks is completely unforgiving if you forget that you are the one that must adjust to it. When accustomed to sneakers on smooth walkways, we can easily forget that we are supposed to be the ones to bend.

Most people walk with far too much tension in their legs. The key to moving less is to begin by softening the legs so that they can bend with ease. Think of the way a toddler can squat down with their back up straight and look at a flower, then think of most older people trying the same action. The difference isn't simply that people are old; it's that they are stiff. With proper training it is possible for an adult to have the same softness and pliability as a child.

SLOW SQUAT AGAINST THE WALL:

Begin with your back against the wall and your legs apart. Start to slowly squat down while sliding against the wall. If you feel tension in your legs, then rise up, take a relaxing breath and shake the tension loose. Repeat the same motion until you can squat down effortlessly. You will find that it is easier to squat down while exhaling smoothly. As you rise up, inhale.

EXERCISE: WIND SHAKES THE TREE

The Chinese say that pain is stagnation: move the stagnation, and the pain goes away. This exercise is designed to remove obstructions and free the body, making it an ideal warm-up. Even people who are bedridden but can move a single finger can use this idea to help keep blood circulating. It also lets you release pent-up energy. When people feel angry, their instinct is to punch, scratch or climb up a tree. This is why their shoulders develop tension when stressed. They hold this tension in their shoulders, which leads to having a stiff neck and a hunched posture.

Fear makes people want to run away. That kind of behavior would cause very awkward social situations. As a result, people hold tension in their legs. This leads to muscle tension associated with joint and back problems. After years of unexpressed tension in the legs, people begin to walk like most elderly people do. To get a new lease on mobility, free yourself of chronic tension by sighing and shaking.

1. Stand with your feet shoulder-width apart and straighten your spine. Imagine that the top of your head is suspended from above and that a weight is pulling your tailbone downward. This visual exercise can help to align the spine. Feel your shoulders hang on your spine and slowly begin shaking your arms. Slow down or stop if you feel pain and work your way into it. The purpose is to

relax and loosen. Continue until you feel a warm sensation spreading over your upper back and shoulders.

2. You can continue shaking your arms, and now begin shaking your legs as though you are scared. Tremble and shake the tension out of your legs. If you feel tension stuck in some part of your leg, breath like you are sighing and let the tension go. Continue to shake your legs until the tension is gone and a warm sensation spreads over your lower back.

3. Stop shaking your arms and legs for a moment and begin bouncing up and down very gently at a low vibration, increasing the frequency and magnitude as you feel comfortable. As you get used to this you can return to shaking your arms and legs as you see fit. Feel yourself get taller as your spine lengthens. This will help to increase communication between your central and peripheral nervous systems and greatly improve your alignment. Continue with this until you get bored.

4. Start to rotate your hips back and forth, beginning slowly and working yourself into a shimmy. Don't try to shake your arms and legs. By moving from the center, your whole body will move by itself.

5. Continue shaking from the waist. Pay attention to the arch of the foot and combine bouncing with shaking. You will notice spirals of force moving through your body. Let them travel through you and move you at will. Have fun with it. If you need inspiration, watch video clips of West African religious ceremonies or go to a Southern Baptist church. Move like that, and you will quickly rid yourself of extra tension. Slow it down and speed it up as needed. Play with the whole range to better understand relaxation and alignment.

LIMITING HEARING:

Get some good earplugs and use them. As you walk, you can hear the internal forces colliding inside yourself. Listen to the sound and begin to adjust your breathing and the softness in your steps until you can't hear yourself walking.

LIMITING VISION:

Try closing your eyes and feeling your steps. Feel your way around using your feel and walk slowly. Create tension in your body and then shift to complete relaxation. Pay attention to how your relative level of tension can blind your movements. Your body uses proprioception to understand where it is in space. Tension can blind this proprioception and make you lose touch with your instinctive movement. By closing off your ears and shutting your eyes, you can get back in touch with these senses.

MOVING AROUND OBSTACLES:

Once you get a feeling for moving without external sound and without visual cues, you can gradually step it up a notch. Scatter obstacles, or have a friend push you or put a leg out to trip you. Move as slowly as possible at first. It should be easy to adjust and move through. Keeping this relaxed feeling, move through the obstacles at an increasingly faster pace. If you feel that you are building up tension, then stop, relax and go at a slower pace.

Eventually, it will be possible to run through a forest

while blindfolded or to adjust to the movements of a group of people who are pushing, pulling and attempting to trip you with fluidity and grace. The concept behind this training is simple enough for people who can barely walk and yet challenging enough for high-level athletes. The only difference is the intensity of the action that will dictate your internal softness. This kind of training is what wild animals live with. They can't turn their head and look at every branch; they need to feel their way through the forest. For their whole lives they learn to move at night and in the rain. They discover how to move with softness and grace to soften the world around them. The world of human society is comfortable and soft. This softness can make people stiff and hard. As the world around us yields, we don't need to be soft. As we become stiffer earlier, we begin aging and lose our natural athleticism. By using external challenges and providing ourselves with a harder environment, it helps us to regain the softness we are supposed to have. This is the essence of unlocking natural athleticism.

EXERCISES FOR THE LONG RUN

If you look at warrior and hunting traditions from around the world, you will find an approach to athleticism that is functional and results in long-term joint health. These traditions do not tend to revolve around isolated strength so much as mental attitude, tensegrity and alignment. Tensegrity is how your body works together as a unit. Think of the way a cat moves and contrast it to the way a bodybuilder moves. The cat moves with fluidity and grace, whereas the bodybuilder trains for isolated contraction. Cats are among nature's best hunters. The way they move makes them resistant to extreme forces, giving the impression that they have nine lives.

If you want to live long and enjoy healthy joints, make yourself as soft and poised as a cat. The heavier you are, the stronger the forces are that travel through your body. The waves of force created by taking a single step can generate forces several times your body weight. If the force does not travel evenly through you, it collides internally, causing joint damage. To understand how the forces begin in our feet and travel through the body, it's important to start from the ground up.

THE TENSEGRITY ARCH

Your foot contains hundreds of integrated arches. The

whole of the foot forms something of a dome. It is an incredible design for distributing force. The arch is one of the greatest engineering marvels ever created; Roman bridges still stand as a testament to this incredible structure. The human body is engineered in a similar way. The two legs form an arch, the armpits also provide arches if you are walking on all fours. The sacrum and pelvis are filled with arches and circles to make the human skeleton as strong and lightweight as possible. You are capable of distributing incredible forces, thanks to the arches which permeate our structure.

Tensegrity arches create a fluid structure throughout your body. Your pelvis is a circle. The sacrum has smaller circles and our joints are likewise circular. You are composed of arches and overlapping circular distributions of force that spiral and travel in waves throughout your body. The spine, rather than being a column, is snakelike and can be supported by muscle independently of gravity. You have several different types of connective tissue and muscle that not only help you to hold a position, but also make you flexible enough to distribute incredible forces.

Your feet act as feelers to maintain a fluid alignment

throughout the body. Seven thousand nerve endings in each human foot communicate with the rest of the body. They also play a role in blood circulation and keep motion traveling smoothly through you. The foot is to your physical structure what your tongue is to your digestion. Your feet serve as sensors. As your foot bends in one direction, a chain reaction moves through the entire body. Overly padded shoes do little to stop the impact, but they do serve to blind your feet. The end result is that you are taking forces at up to ten times your body weight with only an inch of padding to save you. This sends a zigzag shockwave to your ankles, knees, lumbar vertebrae and neck, and is particularly problematic if you have extra weight and reduced circulation, making it harder for damaged joints to heal.

This is why many people don't feel like exercising; it isn't laziness so much as intelligence. Imagine getting smashed with a baseball bat at forces up to ten times your body weight. Even with an inch of padding around the bat, it wouldn't take long before you might prefer a sedentary lifestyle. Your true shock absorbers are not the padding in your shoes or your cartilage; rather, you are not designed to bounce on these things while moving with stiff legs. You are designed to have shockwaves travel freely through you.

Footsteps make sounds. The worse you are walking, the noisier your footsteps become. If you are making a lot of noise while walking, then you are causing internal damage. Walk softly. Breathe softly. Human beings are hidden foragers and silent killers. The way we evolved to hunt, forage and survive is based on silence. The foundation of this stealth and endurance is relaxation. The secret behind efficient movement is that there is no replacement for good movement. With the correct movement, bare feet are sufficient for running. With the wrong technique, expensive shoes won't save you – it doesn't matter how many springs, air pockets or doodads they add.

In *Born to Run*, Christopher McDougall sheds light on the modern myth of running shoes. He writes, "Until 1972, when the modern athletic shoe was invented, people ran in very thin-soled shoes, had strong feet and had a much lower incidence of knee injuries."

Dr. Daniel Lieberman, professor of biological anthropology at Harvard University, has been studying the growing injury crisis in the developed world for some time and has come to a startling conclusion: "A lot of foot and knee injuries currently plaguing us are caused by people running with shoes that actually make our feet weak, cause us to over-pronate (ankle rotation) and give us knee problems."

Don't throw out your sneakers just yet, though. Until the feet are strong enough, the support will be necessary. According to Michael McCourt, a podiatrist in Eugene, Oregon, being overweight can cause increased ankle pronation. He explains that being overweight causes anterior pelvic tilt, otherwise known as. In addition, carrying more weight requires people to have a 30 percent wider stance. Given the angle, this makes heavier people more susceptible to over-pronation. If a person's stance is already compromised, it makes no sense to begin running or doing squats when proper alignment will be all but impossible to achieve.

The first step is to perfect the arch and strengthen it slowly. Most city blocks in China house at least one foot-massage clinic. In fact, this is the most prevalent use of Chinese medicine in China. It is a matter of practicality rather than luxury. If your ankle, knee and spine problems are massaged and cracked into place, what use is it if every step undermines your treatment? It makes more sense to work first with your foundation.

Many people find relief from complex alignment issues through foot soaks and massage. You begin by soaking your feet in a hot herbal infusion to improve circulation, soften the feet, and reduce inflammation. Then you get a rather intense massage. Each of those seven thousand nerves in the foot will be singing. Your feet suddenly seem like two living fish instead of chunks of ice. The joints of your foot move in ways you never thought possible. You get up, take a few steps, and your back pain feels better. This is mainly because the treatment has reestablished your body's primary feeler and shock absorber. When the foot is communicating with the rest of the body, the arches distribute forces up and through the body in a series of fluid spirals rather than slamming into your joints and crushing your bones against one another. A lot of chronic pain comes down to stiff feet.

EXERCISE: FOOT MASSAGE

Start by soaking your feet in warm water for 15–20 minutes, and increase the temperature until your veins are bulging out and your foot begins to soften. Your blood vessels will relax and expand due to nitric oxide, and your blood will start transferring the heat evenly throughout your body. The fresh blood nourishes, heals, and softens the foot.

This same process helps to regulate the distribution of nitric oxide, which can burn fat, balance the gut microbiome and alleviate pain.

Once your feet are soft, you can have a friend massage them. If you don't have someone who can help massage your feet, then put some smooth rocks into the bucket. As you sit, you can press downward on the rocks for an easy massage.[18]

EXERCISE: STACKING BONES VISUALIZATION

First, imagine the various bones of your foot and how they feel. Pay attention to the weight distribution. Visualize the bones of your foot and slowly build your structure from the ground up. Think of it like stacking blocks and adjust your posture accordingly. If you are sitting down, think of your pelvis and lumbar spine and adjust your posture so that you require minimal force to maintain your posture. Begin by doing this throughout the day from a position of stillness. Later, as you move around, continue using this visualization to help maintain your stability.

---

[18] *Use smooth stones and common sense. 24 – Credit to Jerry Alan Johnson DMQ*

MARIONETTE

Imagine that your head is suspended from above and pulled upward like a marionette, and that a weight is on your tailbone pulling downward. This is a common visualization in Chinese martial arts used to help people find relaxation and alignment.

ADJUSTING BALANCE

Long-term fitness begins with alignment and gentle movement. Before you begin running and jumping, you should ensure that you have good alignment. This is how you release the waves of motion to travel freely throughout body, making the act of moving more like a massage than a beating.

EXERCISE: WATERFALL MEDITATION

This is a visualization for relaxing and aligning the body.

1. Begin standing with your legs shoulder-width apart, with your hands hanging freely at your sides. Imagine a waterfall coming from above, washing over your body and down the sides of your arms and legs. Visualize it cleaning, relaxing, soothing

and filling you with this heavenly water. Imagine the water running over you. Continue this for 5 minutes.

2. Next, imagine that this water is running down the front of your body. Continue for five minutes.

3. Visualize the water flowing down the back of your legs. Continue for five minutes.

4. Visualize water flowing through you, exiting the bottoms of your feet and through your pores. Imagine it washing you completely, freeing you of tension and aligning your body.

THE WAVES WITHIN

One of my earliest memories is watching my grandfather find a stud in the wall for a remodeling project. He knocked along the wall listening for a change in resonance and easily located the studs. It's a simple technique you have used before, the same way you might knock on a basin of water to determine how full it is. The exercises outlined in this book are largely based on this same idea. If you have followed the exercises so far, you have already started to study waves of motion. You have felt intestinal waves as food moved through your digestive tract. As you develop deeper relaxation, it is common to feel pulsing in the spine. This is your cerebrospinal fluid pump. You can feel this providing your brain with healthy circulation. When you achieve this level of sensitivity, it is not unusual to feel sensations of heat traveling through the body. This is the effect of gases such as nitric oxide activating energy and converting fat into heat. If you feel the flow of these waves getting blocked, relax and use the feeling of the obstruction to improve your relaxation and tensegrity. Think of it like using a garden hose. As a kid, I would have water fights that sometimes involved using a hose. The trick to winning a water fight against someone with a hose was to put a kink in it to obstruct the flow. Once the flow of water stopped, I had two choices. I could either run over to unkink it and lose my position at the nozzle, or I could send a wave rippling through the hose to release the flow. It didn't take long to figure out that using a wave is much easier than trying to go over and manually unkink the hose. This is an important lesson to remember about the human body. It is filled with fluids, gases and pathways that benefit from these same wavelike motions.

Think of a river. As the water flows over a rock, you can see the wave rise above it. In a still pond, a pebble disturbing the surface will cause a ripple that will continue outward until it hits something solid, and then the vibration will reflect backwards. Similarly, as waves travel through your body, you can feel for areas of tension. Use large waves and shorter waves and alter the frequency and pitch of the vibrations to find areas of hidden tension. As you begin to loosen up, your body will seek an efficient alignment. It is normal to feel some slight tension keeping you out of alignment. You may notice certain muscle groups pulling your body toward the unhealthy postures you might be accustomed to. For those who sit down a lot, the hip flexors tend to be tense, while the abdominal muscles are loose. This tips your hips forward and brings your tailbone back into a posture called lordosis, which causes undue strain on the knees and lumbar spine. Everyone has a different lifestyle and unique ways of moving. There are times when you are in a state of poor posture and your body learns to hold these positions. As you return to your natural poise, you will discover that some areas may be too tense, while others are too slack. Once you reveal these areas to yourself, you can then stretch them or strengthen them depending on what you need.

EXERCISE: WIND SHAKES THE TREE

See Page 242.

EXERCISE: MASTERING MOVEMENT FOR OPTIMUM ATHLETICISM

Whether you are an elite athlete or simply trying to walk without pain, this exercise is very important. It is based on the same idea of relaxing, freeing up energy and reinvesting it.

1. Consider how waves of force move through you. If they get stuck at any points, use breathing to smooth the waves of force and relax the tension until most of the energy is flowing through you freely.

2. Now that you have free forces moving through you, look at how you can use them. If you are walking, use the upward spiral to move your next foot forward.

3. Discover how much force is required to move you

from one motion to the next. Recycle one motion into another. If extra forces are moving out of your head or extending through your body, then focus on the distribution of force. Use only the minimum effort to move freely and smoothly. Getting the body to work smoothly as a relaxed whole is more important than isolated motion.

4. Now begin adding more power. Increase your force until it no longer feels smooth, then repeat steps 1–3. Continue until you can increase the forces you generate. As you increase force, you will notice that some of the force gets trapped or leaks outward from the joints. Adjust your structure as you add resistance until the forces can comfortably travel through your structure.

STILLNESS AND MOTION

Balance stillness and motion. Motion can help your circulation to move outward and stillness can draw it inward toward your internal organs for healing and repair. Stillness exercises include meditation and relaxation techniques that cause you to feel rested and powered up. More dynamic exercises include running, jumping, swimming, hiking and activities that can make you feel tired. Use both rest and movement in order to heal yourself and make yourself stronger.

Lu Zijian was a strong proponent of using stillness and motion for health. He was born in 1893 and began learning martial arts from his mother. Later he went to study under several notable masters. In 1920, he won the gold medal at the Nanjing Yuhuatai martial arts competition. Later, Chiang Kaishek, leader of the Kuomintang, appointed him to general and commissioned him to train his personal bodyguards.

Lu Zijian established a martial arts school and a famous clinic of Chinese medicine where he helped generations of people find health and balance in their lives. If you want to see an exceptional athlete moving like a cat at over 100 years of age, you can find YouTube videos of him performing martial arts and even doing a somersault while holding swords. Before he passed on at the age of 118, he gave the following advice:

"Move your qi, nurture your health and cultivate your nature. Training martial arts will make your limbs agile.

Exercise using moving and stillness. This is the correct method to reach a long life."

Stillness

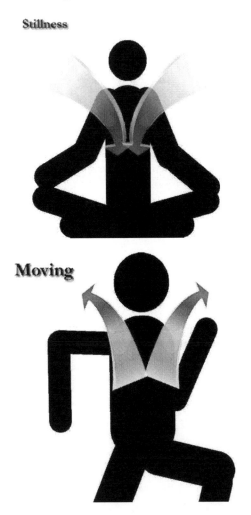

Moving

MOVEMENT COVERS A MULTITUDE OF DIETARY SINS

When you start moving, it automatically begins to alter your food cravings. If you eat junk food and then start moving, you will probably feel nauseous. If you are moving every day, then every time you eat something inappropriate and start moving, you will begin notice physiological differences in your body. The harder you exercise, the more obvious these feelings become. Your body will tell you what it needs, but only if you are moving and listening to it. The stronger you become, the less your diet really matters. The free flow of gasotransmitters will tend your garden of life. Your gut will automatically give you very strong feeding signals to only eat appropriate foods. At this point you are in sync with your gut microbiota and they are taking care of the details so that you don't have to think about it.

BALANCE BLOOD FLOW

Generally speaking, the night is colder than the day and winter is cooler than summer. The cooler weather causes blood to be directed to your internal organs where it can protect and nourish them. Because of this, it is easier to do exercises for the internal organs in winter. Still, to avoid extremes, you want to stay active so that you maintain peripheral blood circulation. A good way to do this is to do some dynamic exercises to warm up in winter and then begin meditation as the major focus in your training.

In warmer weather, blood goes to the exterior of the body where it can release heat and cool the body. This makes dynamic physical exercise easier during the day and in the summer. To avoid extremes, direct some of your effort internally through meditation, balance or alignment exercises. This makes a nice warm-up and cool-down for more intense athletic activity.

Chapter 18: The Road to a Pain Free Life

Step 1. Discovery

1. Begin with the quiz (see Fibrobible.com or Fibrocircle.com). Discover which type of fibromyalgia is predominant .

2. Determine what your strategy of care will be.

3. Realistically apply it to your schedule.

Step 2. The branches of pain

The first major step for alleviating fibromyalgia pains to regulate the flow of gasotransmitters. This is best done through qigong and acupuncture. In order for this to be successful, consistency is key. In North America many people will do qigong or acupuncture once a week. As a result of this under dosing the results are often limited. In China qigong is practiced up to 3 times a day and acupuncture is done daily or every other day. This allows for fast pain relief because once the distribution is well regulated, the pain will stop. At this stage many people believe they are done with their healing process, but in actuality, they are only halfway there. Many people with fibromyalgia will find something that works for a while, but not in the long run. This is because it is affecting their levels of inflammation in the short run, but not addressing the deeper imbalances of the endocrine system.

Step 3: The hidden roots

The third step when addressing fibromyalgia is to regulate the gut. As the gut-brain axis comes back under control it becomes easier to sleep better. As sleep improves the underlying regulatory systems of the hypothalamus-pituitary-adrenal axis begin to return to a health rhythm. When sustained with a healthy lifestyle people find that their fibromyalgia symptoms leave and never return.

CONTINUING THE CYCLE

This is a process of learning about the world using your own physical experience. It's the study of life within you and understanding at a physical level how connected you are to the world around you. These physical experiences occur both in motion and at rest. With the right perspective, you can make use of everything. What's important is that you are learning about yourself and how you fit into the world that surrounds you. This is ultimately the way to beat fibromyalgia and live a great life.

As you turn with the seasons, you will better understand how to master your microbiome and the world will become your garden, your pharmacy and your playground.

As long as you breathe, the forces of nature will affect you. The wind will blow, the road will turn and you will get jostled about. Mean people will exist and contribute to your emotional fluctuations. You will ingest poison, make mistakes and fall down from time to time. This is all part of life. As your microbiome shifts with the seasonal cycles, you can learn more about nature and about yourself. Your internal garden isn't grown in a day. Like any garden, it requires observation, tending and time.

Pay attention to these cycles and reconnect with your instincts. With this simple change in perspective, you will begin to discover how to master the rhythms with every step, every breath, every birth and every death. As you harmonize your internal world with the environment, you will return at last to paradise.

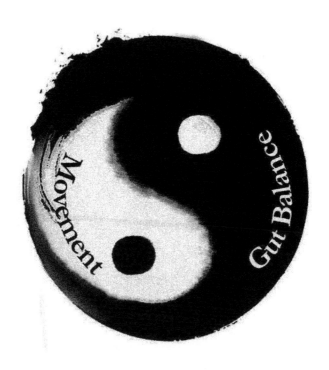

RECAP:

To warm and dry: Pungent, bland and bitter foods combined with sweating and breathing as though you are yawning.

To warm and moisten: Pungent, salty, sweet and oily foods combined with breathing like you are yawning.

To cool and moisten: Sour and salty foods combined with sighing breaths. More sedentary internal exercises which draw blood circulation inward.

To cool and dry: Sour and bitter foods combined with sighing breaths. More stomach massage or other exercises that increase bowel movements and urination.

Use both movement and rest to your advantage. Relax, stand up straight, and if something is stuck, use a wave to free it. That's it. Enjoy.

References

1. Varela, Mariana, Thomas E. Spencer, Massimo Palmarini, and Frederick Arnaud. "Friendly viruses." *Annals of the New York Academy of Sciences* 1178, no. 1 (2009): 157-172.

2. Ramakrishna, Balakrishnan S. "The normal bacterial flora of the human intestine and its regulation." *Journal of clinical gastroenterology* 41 (2007): S2-S6.

3. Niess, Jan Hendrik, Frank Leithäuser, Guido Adler, and Jörg Reimann. "Commensal gut flora drives the expansion of proinflammatory CD4 T cells in the colonic lamina propria under normal and inflammatory conditions." *The Journal of Immunology* 180, no. 1 (2008): 559-568.

4. Thompson, Jeffrey M., et al. "Direct medical costs in patients with fibromyalgia: cost of illness and impact of a brief multidisciplinary treatment program." *American Journal of Physical Medicine & Rehabilitation* 90.1 (2011): 40-46.

5. Kluger, MATTHEW J., CAROLE A. Conn, B. R. E. N. D. A. Franklin, R. O. L. F. Freter, and GERALD D. Abrams. "Effect of gastrointestinal flora on body temperature of rats and mice." *American Journal of Physiology-Regulatory, Integrative and Comparative Physiology* 258, no. 2 (1990): R552-R557.

6. Klaus, Susanne, Heike Münzberg, Christiane Trüloff, and Gerhard Heldmaier. "Physiology of transgenic mice with brown fat ablation: obesity is due to lowered body temperature." *American Journal of Physiology-Regulatory, Integrative and Comparative Physiology* 274, no. 2 (1998): R287-R293.

7. Hoffman, Lucas R., David A. D'Argenio, Michael J. MacCoss, Zhaoying Zhang, Roger A. Jones, and Samuel I. Miller. "Aminoglycoside antibiotics induce bacterial biofilm formation." *Nature* 436, no. 7054 (2005): 1171-1175.

8. Karatan, Ece, and Paula Watnick. "Signals, regulatory networks, and materials that build and break bacterial biofilms." *Microbiology and Molecular Biology Reviews* 73, no. 2 (2009): 310-347.

9. Cani, Patrice D., and Nathalie M. Delzenne. "Interplay between obesity and associated metabolic disorders: new insights into the gut microbiota." *Current opinion in pharmacology 9*, no. 6 (2009): 737-743.

10. Turnbaugh, Peter J., and Jeffrey I. Gordon. "The core gut microbiome, energy balance and obesity." *The Journal of physiology* 587, no. 17 (2009): 4153-4158.

11. Li, Kelvin, Monika Bihan, Shibu Yooseph, and Barbara A. Methé. "Analyses of the microbial diversity across the human microbiome." *PLoS One* 7, no. 6 (2012): e32118.

12. Grabitske, Hollie A., and Joanne L. Slavin. "Gastrointestinal effects of low-digestible carbohydrates." *Critical reviews in food science and nutrition* 49, no. 4 (2009): 327-360.

13. De Filippo, Carlotta, et al. "Impact of diet in shaping gut microbiota revealed by a comparative study in children from Europe and rural Africa." *Proceedings of the National Academy of Sciences* 107.33 (2010): 14691-14696.

14. Gershon, Michael D. *The second brain.* HarperCollins Publishers, 1998.

15. Cerqueira, Fernanda M., Fernanda M. da Cunha, Camille C. Caldeira da Silva, Bruno Chausse, Renato L. Romano, Camila Garcia, Pio Colepicolo, Marisa HG Medeiros, and Alicia J. Kowaltowski. "Long-term intermittent feeding, but not caloric restriction, leads to redox imbalance, insulin receptor nitration, and glucose intolerance." *Free Radical Biology and Medicine* 51, no. 7 (2011): 1454-1460.

16. Mestdagh, Renaud, Marc-Emmanuel Dumas, Serge Rezzi, Sunil Kochhar, Elaine Holmes, Sandrine P. Claus, and Jeremy K. Nicholson. "Gut microbiota modulate the metabolism of brown adipose tissue in mice." *Journal of proteome research* 11, no. 2 (2011): 620-630.

17. Maes, Michael, Marta Kubera, Jean-Claude Leunis, and Michael Berk. "Increased IgA and IgM responses against gut commensals in chronic depression: further evidence for

increased bacterial translocation or leaky gut."*Journal of affective disorders* 141, no. 1 (2012): 55-62.

18. Duncan, S. H., G. E. Lobley, G. Holtrop, J. Ince, A. M. Johnstone, P. Louis, and H. J. Flint. "Human colonic microbiota associated with diet, obesity and weight loss." *International journal of obesity* 32, no. 11 (2008): 1720-1724.

19. Zupancic, Margaret L., Brandi L. Cantarel, Zhenqiu Liu, Elliott F. Drabek, Kathleen A. Ryan, Shana Cirimotich, Cheron Jones et al. "Analysis of the gut microbiota in the old order Amish and its relation to the metabolic syndrome."*PLoS One* 7, no. 8 (2012): e43052.

20. Ishimaru, Yoshiro, Hitoshi Inada, Momoka Kubota, Hanyi Zhuang, Makoto Tominaga, and Hiroaki Matsunami. "Transient receptor potential family members PKD1L3 and PKD2L1 form a candidate sour taste receptor."*Proceedings of the National Academy of Sciences* 103, no. 33 (2006): 1256912574.

21. Collins, Stephen M., Michael Surette, and Premysl Bercik. "The interplay between the intestinal microbiota and the brain." *Nature Reviews Microbiology* 10, no. 11 (2012): 735

22. Cryan, John F., and Timothy G. Dinan. "Mind-altering microorganisms: the impact of the gut microbiota on brain and behaviour." *Nature Reviews Neuroscience* 13, no. 10 (2012): 701-712.

23. Costandi, Moheb. "Microbes on Your Mind." *Scientific American Mind* 23, no. 3 (2012): 32-37.

24. Neufeld, K. M., N. Kang, J. Bienenstock, and J. A. Foster. "Reduced anxiety-like behavior and central neurochemical change in germ-free mice."*Neurogastroenterology & Motility* 23, no. 3 (2011): 255-e119.

25. Kallmeyer, Jens, Robert Pockalny, Rishi Ram Adhikari, David C. Smith, and Steven D'Hondt. "Global distribution of microbial abundance and biomass in subseafloor sediment." *Proceedings of the National Academy of Sciences* 109, no. 40 (2012): 16213-16216.

26. Luo, Y. H., and W. Y. Zhu. "The intestinal microbiota and

obesity of the host."*Wei sheng wu xue bao= Acta microbiologica Sinica* 47, no. 6 (2007): 1115-1118.

27. Ferraris MEG, Munõz AC. Histología y embriología bucodental. 3. ed. 2009

28. Edgar, W. M. "Saliva: its secretion, composition and functions." *British dental journal* 172, no. 8 (1992): 305-312.

29. Craigen, Bradford, Aliza Dashiff, and Daniel E. Kadouri. "The use of commercially available alpha-amylase compounds to inhibit and remove Staphylococcus aureus biofilms." *The open microbiology journal* 5 (2011): 21.

30. Humphrey, Sue P., and Russell T. Williamson. "A review of saliva: normal composition, flow, and function." *The Journal of prosthetic dentistry* 85, no. 2 (2001): 162-169.

31. Enberg, Nina, Hannu Alho, Vuokko Loimaranta, and Marianne Lenander-Lumikari. "Saliva flow rate, amylase activity, and protein and electrolyte concentrations in saliva after acute alcohol consumption." *Oral Surgery, Oral Medicine, Oral Pathology, Oral Radiology, and Endodontology* 92, no. 3 (2001): 292-298.

32. de Oliveira CG, Collares EF, Barbieri MA, Fernandes MIM. "Produção e concentração de saliva e amilase salivar em crianças obesas.: *Arq Gastroenterol*. 1997, 34:105-111.

33. Ten Cate AR. Oral Histology: Development, Structure and Function. 5th ed. St. Louis: Mosby; 1998

34. Kerti, Lucia, A. Veronica Witte, Angela Winkler, Ulrike Grittner, Dan Rujescu, and Agnes Flöel. "Higher glucose levels associated with lower memory and reduced hippocampal microstructure." *Neurology* 81, no. 20 (2013): 1746-1752.

35. Bercik, Premysl, Emmanuel Denou, Josh Collins, Wendy Jackson, Jun Lu, Jennifer Jury, Yikang Deng et al. "The intestinal microbiota affect central levels of brain-derived neurotropic factor and behavior in mice." *Gastroenterology* 141, no. 2 (2011): 599-609.

36. Tannock, G. W. "Effect of dietary and environmental stress on the gastrointestinal microbiota." *Human Intestinal Microflora in*

Health and Disease (1983): 517-539.

37. Flegr, Jaroslav. "Effects of Toxoplasma on human behavior." *Schizophrenia bulletin* 33, no. 3 (2007): 757-760.

38. Zhang, Yuanfen, Lil Traskman-Bendz, Shorena Janelidze, Patricia Langenberg, Ahmed Saleh, Niel Constantine, Olaoluwa Okusaga, Cecilie Bay-Richter, Lena Brundin, and Teodor T. Postolache. "Toxoplasma gondii immunoglobulin G antibodies and nonfatal suicidal self-directed violence." *J Clin psychiatry* 73, no. 8 (2012): 1069-1076.

39. Stack, Kathleen M., and Athena S. Papas. "Xerostomia: etiology and clinical management." *Nutrition in clinical care* 4, no. 1 (2001): 15-21.

40. Amerongen, A. V., and E. C. I. Veerman. "Saliva–the defender of the oral cavity." *Oral diseases* 8, no. 1 (2002): 12-22.

41. Dawes, C. "Circadian rhythms in human salivary flow rate and composition." *The Journal of physiology* 220, no. 3 (1972): 529545.

42. Menifield, Charles E., Nicole Doty, and Audwin Fletcher. "Obesity in America." *ABNF Journal* 19, no. 3 (2008): 83-88.

43. Séralini, Gilles-Eric, Emilie Clair, Robin Mesnage, Steeve Gress, Nicolas Defarge, Manuela Malatesta, Didier Hennequin, and Joël Spiroux de Vendômois. "Long term toxicity of a Roundup herbicide and a Roundup-tolerant genetically modified maize." *Food and Chemical Toxicology* 50, no. 11 (2012): 4221-4231.

44. Ordovas, Jose M., and Vincent Mooser. "Nutrigenomics and nutrigenetics." *Current opinion in lipidology* 15, no. 2 (2004): 101-108.

45. Wooley, C. S., and David M. Garner. "Controversies in management: Dietary treatments for obesity are ineffective." Bmj 309, no. 6955 (1994): 655-656.

46. Grundy, David. "Signalling the state of the digestive tract." *Autonomic Neuroscience* 125, no. 1 (2006): 76-80.

47. Zhang, Yiying, Ricardo Proenca, Margherita Maffei, Marisa Barone, Lori Leopold, and Jeffrey M. Friedman. "Positional cloning of the mouse obese gene and its human homologue."

Nature 372, no. 6505 (1994): 425-432.

48. Niswender, Kevin D., Denis G. Baskin, and Michael W. Schwartz. "Insulin and its evolving partnership with leptin in the hypothalamic control of energy homeostasis." *Trends in Endocrinology & Metabolism* 15, no. 8 (2004): 362-369.

49. Frei, Robert, Claudio Gaucher, Simon W. Poulton, and Don E. Canfield. "Fluctuations in Precambrian atmospheric oxygenation recorded by chromium isotopes." *Nature* 461, no. 7261 (2009): 250-253.

50. Burguera, Bartolome, Marta E. Couce, Geoffry L. Curran, Michael D. Jensen, Ricardo V. Lloyd, Margot P. Cleary, and Joseph F. Poduslo. "Obesity is associated with a decreased leptin transport across the blood-brain barrier in rats." *Diabetes* 49, no. 7 (2000): 1219-1223.

51. Cawley, John, and Chad Meyerhoefer. "The medical care costs of obesity: an instrumental variables approach." *Journal of health economics* 31, no. 1 (2012): 219-230.

52. Wang, Y. Claire, Klim McPherson, Tim Marsh, Steven L. Gortmaker, and Martin Brown. "Health and economic burden of the projected obesity trends in the USA and the UK." *The Lancet* 378, no. 9793 (2011): 815-825.

53. Finucane, Mariel M., Gretchen A. Stevens, Melanie J. Cowan, Goodarz Danaei, John K. Lin, Christopher J. Paciorek, Gitanjali M. Singh et al. "National, regional, and global trends in body-mass index since 1980: systematic analysis of health examination surveys and epidemiological studies with 960 country-years and 9.1 million participants." The Lancet 377, no. 9765 (2011): 557-567.

54. World Health Organization. Obesity and Overweight. Updated March 2013. www.who.int/mediacentre/factsheets/fs311/en/. Accessed on April 29, 2013

55. Wang, Youfa, May A. Beydoun, Lan Liang, Benjamin Caballero, and Shiriki K. Kumanyika. "Will all Americans become overweight or obese? Estimating the progression and cost of the

US obesity epidemic." *Obesity* 16, no. 10 (2008): 2323-2330.

56. Trogdon, J. G., E. A. Finkelstein, T. Hylands, P. S. Dellea, and S. J. Kamal-Bahl. "Indirect costs of obesity: a review of the current literature." *Obesity Reviews* 9, no. 5 (2008): 489-500.

57. Stunkard, Albert J., and Thomas A. Wadden. "Psychological aspects of severe obesity." *The American journal of clinical nutrition* 55, no. 2 (1992): 524S-532S.

58. Harvey, E. L., and A. J. Hill. "Health professionals' views of overweight people and smokers." *International Journal of Obesity & Related Metabolic Disorders* 25, no. 8 (2001).

59. Edwards, Ryan D. "Public transit, obesity, and medical costs: assessing the magnitudes." *Preventive Medicine* 46, no. 1 (2008): 14-21.

60. Björntorp, Per, and Roland Rosmond. "Obesity and cortisol." *Nutrition* 16, no. 10 (2000): 924-936.

61. Skrzypski, M. T. T. L., T. T. Le, P. Kaczmarek, E. Pruszynska-Oszmalek, P. Pietrzak, D. Szczepankiewicz, P. A. Kolodziejski et al. "Orexin A stimulates glucose uptake, lipid accumulation and adiponectin secretion from 3T3-L1 adipocytes and isolated primary rat adipocytes." *Diabetologia* 54, no. 7 (2011): 18411852.

62. Saunders, Travis J., Richard Larouche, Rachel C. Colley, and Mark S. Tremblay. "Acute sedentary behaviour and markers of cardiometabolic risk: a systematic review of intervention studies." *Journal of nutrition and metabolism* 2012 (2012).

63. Benedict, Christian, Manfred Hallschmid, Astrid Hatke, Bernd Schultes, Horst L. Fehm, Jan Born, and Werner Kern. "Intranasal insulin improves memory in humans." *Psychoneuroendocrinology* 29, no. 10 (2004): 1326-1334.

64. Gonzales, Mitzi M., Takashi Tarumi, Steven C. Miles, Hirofumi Tanaka, Furqan Shah, and Andreana P. Haley. "Insulin Sensitivity as a Mediator of the Relationship Between BMI and Working Memory-Related Brain Activation." *Obesity* 18, no. 11 (2010): 2131-2137.

65. Ching, ShiNung, Patrick L. Purdon, Sujith Vijayan, Nancy J. Kopell, and Emery N. Brown. "A neurophysiological–metabolic model for burst suppression." *Proceedings of the National Academy of Sciences* 109, no. 8 (2012): 3095-3100.

66. Behari, J., K. K. Kunjilwar, and S. Pyne. "Interaction of low level modulated RF radiation with Na+–K+-ATPase." *Bioelectrochemistry and Bioenergetics* 47, no. 2 (1998): 247-252.

67. Wurtman, Richard J., and Judith J. Wurtman. "Brain Serotonin, Carbohydrate-Craving, Obesity and Depression." *Obesity Research* 3, no. S4 (1995): 477S-480S.

68. Gustafson, T. B., and D. B. Sarwer. "Childhood sexual abuse and obesity." *Obesity reviews* 5, no. 3 (2004): 129-135.

69. Pimentel, Mark, Henry C. Lin, Pedram Enayati, Brian van den Burg, Hyo-Rang Lee, Jin H. Chen, Sandy Park, Yuthana Kong, and Jeffrey Conklin. "Methane, a gas produced by enteric bacteria, slows intestinal transit and augments small intestinal contractile activity." *American Journal of Physiology-Gastrointestinal and Liver Physiology* 290, no. 6 (2006): G1089-G1095.

70. Basseri, Robert J., Benjamin Basseri, Mark Pimentel, Kelly Chong, Adrienne Youdim, Kimberly Low, Laura Hwang, Edy Soffer, Christopher Chang, and Ruchi Mathur. "Intestinal methane production in obese individuals is associated with a higher body mass index." *Gastroenterology & hepatology* 8, no. 1 (2012): 22.

71. Steffey, Eugene P., Brynte H. Johnson, Edmond I. Eger, and Donald Howland Jr. "Nitrous oxide: effect on accumulation rate and uptake of bowel gases." *Anesthesia & Analgesia* 58, no. 5 (1979): 405-408.

72. Jastreboff, Ania M. "Oxytocin Curbs Cookie Consumption." *Science Translational Medicine* 5, no. 208 (2013): 208ec173-208ec173.

73. Jeong, Seung Uk, and Sung Koo Lee. "Obesity and gallbladder diseases." *The Korean Journal of Gastroenterology* 59, no. 1 (2012): 27-34.

74. Erlinger, Serge. "Gallstones in obesity and weight loss." *European journal of gastroenterology & hepatology* 12, no. 12 (2000): 1347-1352.

75. Yang, Huiying, Gloria M. Petersen, Marie-Paule Roth, Leslie J. Schoenfield, and Jay W. Marks. "Risk factors for gallstone formation during rapid loss of weight." *Digestive diseases and sciences* 37, no. 6 (1992): 912-918.

76. Lee, Hui Cheng, Andrew M. Jenner, Chin Seng Low, and Yuan Kun Lee. "Effect of tea phenolics and their aromatic fecal bacterial metabolites on intestinal microbiota." *Research in microbiology* 157, no. 9 (2006): 876-884.

77. Chiang, Chun-Te, Meng-Shih Weng, Shoei-Yn Lin-Shiau, Kuan-Li Kuo, Yao-Jen Tsai, and Jen-Kun Lin. "Pu-erh tea supplementation suppresses fatty acid synthase expression in the rat liver through downregulating Akt and JNK signalings as demonstrated in human hepatoma HepG2 cells." *Oncology Research Featuring Preclinical and Clinical Cancer Therapeutics* 16, no. 3 (2006): 119-128.

78. Haines, Aubrey L. "The Yellowstone Story: A History of Our First National Park, rev. ed., 2 vols." *Niwot, Colo* 1 (1996): 80-82.

79. Creel, Scott, John A. Winnie, and David Christianson. "Glucocorticoid stress hormones and the effect of predation risk on elk reproduction." *Proceedings of the National Academy of Sciences* 106, no. 30 (2009): 12388-12393.

80. Bangs, Ed. *The reintroduction of gray wolves to Yellowstone National Park and central Idaho: final environmental impact statement.* US Fish and Wildlife Service, Gray Wolf EIS, 1994.

81. Douglas H. Chadwick (June–July 2011). "Keystone Species: How Predators Create Abundance and Stability". *Mother Earth News*.http://www.motherearthnews.com/nature-and-environm ent/keystone-species-zm0z11zrog.aspx#axzz31Wdr22lh. Accessed on May 12th, 2014.

82. Dadachova, Ekaterina, Ruth A. Bryan, Xianchun Huang, Tiffany Moadel, Andrew D. Schweitzer, Philip Aisen, Joshua D.

Nosanchuk, and Arturo Casadevall. "Ionizing radiation changes the electronic properties of melanin and enhances the growth of melanized fungi." *PloS one* 2, no. 5 (2007): e457.

83. Liao, Hui, Linda K. Banbury, and David N. Leach. "Antioxidant activity of 45 Chinese herbs and the relationship with their TCM characteristics." *Evidence-based complementary and alternative medicine* 5, no. 4 (2008): 429-434.

84. HaiHua, Luo, Dong Shu, Zhang Sheng, Li Da, Shi Quan, Zhou Hong, and Kuang ZaoYuan. "Effects of Coptidis Decoction on the intestinal flora of mice." *Journal of Tropical Medicine (Guangzhou)* 9, no. 4 (2009): 369-371.

85. Kuo, Kuan-Li, Meng-Shih Weng, Chun-Te Chiang, Yao-Jen Tsai, Shoei-Yn Lin-Shiau, and Jen-Kun Lin. "Comparative studies on the hypolipidemic and growth suppressive effects of oolong, black, pu-erh, and green tea leaves in rats."Journal of agricultural and food chemistry 53, no. 2 (2005): 480-489.

86. Chen, Jia-Xu, Bo Ji, Zhao-Lin Lu, and Li-Sheng Hu. "Effects of Chai Hu (Radix Burpleuri) containing formulation on plasma β-endorphin, epinephrine and dopamine in patients." *The American journal of Chinese medicine* 33, no. 05 (2005): 737-745.

87. Bo, Ji, Chen Jiaxu, and Lu Zhaolin. "Influence of Xiaoyao Powder on Human Nerve-Endocrine-Immune System." *JOURNAL-BEIJING UNIVERSITY OF TRADITIONAL CHINESE MEDICINE* 26, no. 6 (2003): 68-71.

88. Zeng, ZM. "Treating depression with Xiao Yao San." *Journal of Shandong Univeristy of TCM* 22, no.1 (1998): 34-37.

89. Chunfu, Wu, Li Fengli, Liu Wen, and Xu Yongmeng. "Effect of Xiao Yao San on the Levels of Monoamine Neurotransmittres in Rat Brain [J]." *Pharmacology and Clinics of Chinese Materia Medica* 2 (1993): 002.

90. Heinrichs, S. C., and D. Richard. "The role of corticotropin-releasing factor and urocortin in the modulation of ingestive behavior." *Neuropeptides* 33, no. 5 (1999): 350-359.

91. Wang, Shao-Xian, Jia-Xu Chen, Guang-Xin Yue, Ming-Hua Bai,

Mei-Jing Kou, and Zhong-Ye Jin. "Xiaoyaosan decoction regulates changes in neuropeptide Y and leptin receptor in the rat arcuate nucleus after chronic immobilization stress." *Evidence-Based Complementary and Alternative Medicine* 2012 (2012).

92. Chen, J. X., and Y. T. Tang. "Effect of Xiaoyao powder on changes of relative brain zone CRF gene expression in chronic restrained stress rats." *Chinese journal of applied physiology* 20, no. 1 (2004): 71-74.

93. Mizowaki, Maho, Kazuo Toriizuka, and Toshihiko Hanawa. "Anxiolytic effect of Kami-Shoyo-San (TJ-24) in mice possible mediation of neurosteroid synthesis." *Life Sciences* 69, no. 18 (2001): 2167-2177.

94. Bellometti, S., and L. Galzigna. "Function of the hypothalamic adrenal axis in patients with fibromyalgia syndrome undergoing mud-pack treatment." *International journal of clinical pharmacology research* 19, no. 1 (1998): 27-33.

95. Niu, C. S., C. T. Chen, L. J. Chen, K. C. Cheng, C. H. Yeh, and J. T. Cheng. "Decrease of blood lipids induced by Shan-Zha (fruit of Crataegus pinnatifida) is mainly related to an increase of PPARα in liver of mice fed high-fat diet." *Hormone and metabolic research* 43, no. 9 (2011): 625.

96. Gillman, M. A., and F. J. Lichtigfeld. "A comparison of the effects of morphine sulphate and nitrous oxide analgesia on chronic pain states in man." *Journal of the neurological sciences* 49, no. 1 (1981): 41-45.

97. Gillman, M. A., and F. J. Lichtigfeld. "Nitrous oxide interacts with opioid receptors: more evidence." *Anesthesiology* 58, no. 5 (1983): 483.

98. Gillman, MarkA. "Nitrous oxide as neurotransmitter." *The Lancet* 339, no. 8788 (1992): 307.

99. Vizi, E. Sylvester. "Nitric oxide in neurotransmission." *Trends in Pharmacological Sciences* 22, no. 11 (2001): 595.

100. Gillman, M. A. "Discovery of gasotransmission." *SCIENTIST* 18, no. 20 (2004): 10-10.

101. Kinsella, John P., Gary R. Cutter, William F. Walsh, Dale R. Gerstmann, Carl L. Bose, Claudia Hart, Kris C. Sekar et al. "Early inhaled nitric oxide therapy in premature newborns with respiratory failure." *New England Journal of Medicine* 355, no. 4 (2006): 354-364.

102. Dweik, Raed A., Daniel Laskowski, Husam M. Abù-Soud, F. Kaneko, Richard Hutte, Dennis J. Stuehr, and Serpil C. Erzurum. "Nitric oxide synthesis in the lung. Regulation by oxygen through a kinetic mechanism." *Journal of Clinical Investigation* 101, no. 3 (1998): 660.

103. Ballard, Roberta A., William E. Truog, Avital Cnaan, Richard J. Martin, Philip L. Ballard, Jeffrey D. Merrill, Michele C. Walsh et al. "Inhaled nitric oxide in preterm infants undergoing mechanical ventilation." *New England Journal of Medicine* 355, no. 4 (2006): 343-353.

104. Gariaev, Peter, Boris I. Birshtein, Alexander M. Iarochenko, Peter J. Marcer, George G. Tertishny, Katherine A. Leonova, and Uwe Kaempf. "The DNA-wave biocomputer." In *The fourth international conference on computing anticipatory systems* (CASYS), Liege. 2000.

105. Rahnama, Majid, Jack A. Tuszynski, Istvan Bokkon, Michal Cifra, Peyman Sardar, and Vahid Salari. "Emission of mitochondrial biophotons and their effect on electrical activity of membrane via microtubules." *Journal of integrative neuroscience* 10, no. 01 (2011): 65-88.

106. Srilatha, Balasubramanian, Paulpandi Muthulakshmi, P. Ganesan Adaikan, and Philip K. Moore. "Endogenous hydrogen sulfide insufficiency as a predictor of sexual dysfunction in aging rats." *The Aging Male* 15, no. 3 (2012): 153-158.

107. Saha, Shyamal Kumar, and Akihiro Kuroshima. "Nitric oxide and thermogenic function of brown adipose tissue in rats." *The Japanese journal of physiology* 50, no. 3 (2000): 337-342.

108. Jobgen, Wenjuan Shi, Susan K. Fried, Wenjiang J. Fu, Cynthia J. Meininger, and Guoyao Wu. "Regulatory role for the arginine–nitric oxide pathway in metabolism of energy substrates." *The Journal of nutritional biochemistry* 17, no. 9 (2006): 571-588.

109. Wagner, Carsten A. "Hydrogen sulfide: a new gaseous signal molecule and blood pressure regulator." *Journal of nephrology* 22, no. 2 (2008): 173-176.

110. Guzik, T., R. Korbut, and T. Adamek-Guzik. "Nitric oxide and superoxide in inflammation." *Journal of physiology and pharmacology* 54 (2003): 469-487.

111. Giulivi, Cecilia, Juan José Poderoso, and Alberto Boveris. "Production of nitric oxide by mitochondria." *Journal of Biological Chemistry* 273, no. 18 (1998): 11038-11043.

112. Dai, Zhaolai, Zhenlong Wu, Ying Yang, Junjun Wang, M. Carey Satterfield, Cynthia J. Meininger, Fuller W. Bazer, and Guoyao Wu. "Nitric oxide and energy metabolism in mammals." *BioFactors* 39, no. 4 (2013): 383-391.

113. Gupta, S. A. N. D. E. E. P., C. L. A. U. D. I. E. McARTHUR, C. H. R. I. S. T. I. N. E. Grady, and NEIL B. Ruderman. "Stimulation of vascular Na (+)-K (+)-ATPase activity by nitric oxide: a cGMP-independent effect." *American Journal of Physiology-Heart and Circulatory Physiology* 266, no. 5 (1994): H2146-H2151.

114. Ma, Sheng-Xing. "Enhanced nitric oxide concentrations and expression of nitric oxide synthase in acupuncture points/meridians." *The Journal of Alternative & Complementary Medicine* 9, no. 2 (2003): 207-215.

115. Dawson, MD, Ph. D, Ted M., and Valina L. Dawson, Ph. D. "Nitric oxide synthase: role as a transmitter/mediator in the brain and endocrine system." *Annual review of medicine* 47, no. 1 (1996): 219-227.

116. Takehara, Yoshiki, Tomoko Kanno, Tamotsu Yoshioka, Masayasu Inoue, and Kozo Utsumi. "Oxygen-dependent regulation of mitochondrial energy metabolism by nitric oxide." *Archives of biochemistry and biophysics* 323, no. 1 (1995): 27-32.

117. Dotta, B. T., K. S. Saroka, and Michael A. Persinger. "Increased photon emission from the head while imagining light in the dark is correlated with changes in electroencephalographic power: Support for Bókkon's Biophoton Hypothesis." *Neuroscience letters* 513, no. 2 (2012): 151-154.

118. May, Petra, Estelle Woldt, Rachel L. Matz, and Philippe Boucher. "The LDL receptor-related protein (LRP) family: an old family of proteins with new physiological functions." *Annals of medicine* 39, no. 3 (2007): 219-228.

119. Lin, Qiushi, and Jidi Chen. "Molecular mechanism of hawthorn and its flavonoids in prevention on lipid metabolism disorder in rats." [Ying yang xue bao] *Acta nutrimenta Sinica* 22, no. 2 (1999): 131-136.

120. Ying, Gao, and Xiao Ying. "Effect of hawthorn and hawthorn flavonoids extract on rats with hyperlipidemia [J]." *Chinese Journal of Food Hygiene* 3 (2002): 003.

121. Duan, F.J. Prescriptions of Chinese Materia Medica. *ShangHai Scientific and Technological Literature Publishing House*, 1998, Shanghai, China

122. 121.LIU, Guo-sheng, Li LI, Yu-guang DUAN, Liang WANG, Wei-mei ZHANG, and Shi-shu HAO. "Effects of Hawthorn Extracts Isolated by Different Polar Solvent on Blood Fat and

Hemorheological Indexes in Rats with Hyperlipidemia [J]."*Journal of Anhui Traditional Chinese Medical College* 1 (2008): 015.

123. Wu, S.J., Li Q.J., Xiao, XF, Li, M., Yang, X.R., Li, T. "Research on Chemical Components and Pharmacology of Shan Zha." *Drug Evaluation Research* (2010): 316-319.

124. Jun, Li, and Feng Jun. "An Outline Introduction on Dual Pharmacological Effects of Antihypertension and Concurrently Antihyperlipemia of Solo Chinese Medicinal Herbs [J]." *ShiZhen Journal of Traditional Chinese Medicine Research* 1 (1997).

125. LI, Min, Tuo-ping LI, Jun-wei ZHANG, Feng-wen YAN, Zhong-sheng ZHAO, Hui-sheng YAN, and Na WANG. "Antimicrobial activity of essential oil from haw seed." *Science and Technology of Food Industry* 12 (2010): 019.

126. Weng, Y.L. "Pharmacology of Shan Zha." *China Pharmaceutics* 4 (2005): 89-90.

127. Chen, L., Chen, H.P., Liu, Y.P., Hu, Y. "Pharmacological Action of Different Part of Fructus Mume." *China Pharmacy* 18 (2007): 2089-2090

128. Ruan Y.M. "Review of Chemical Components and Pharmacological Actions of Wu Mei." *Chinese Journal of Medicinal Guide* 10 (2008): 793-794

129. 128.Chen H.P., Chen L., Liu Y.P., Hu Y. "Analysis of Fatty Oil of Different Part of Fructus Mume." *Lishizhen Medicine and Materia Medica Research* 18 (2007): 2106-2107

130. Liu Y.P., Chen H.P., Wan D.G., Yan Z.Y., Chen L. "Research Progress of Wu Mei." *Journal of Chinese Medicinal Materials* 27 (2004): 459-462

131. Lee, Hui-Young, Jong-Hwan Park, Seung-Hyeok Seok,

Min-Won Baek, Dong-Jae Kim, Ki-Eun Lee, Kyung-Soo Paek, Yeonhee Lee, and Jae-Hak Park. "Human originated bacteria, Lactobacillus rhamnosus PL60, produce conjugated linoleic acid and show anti-obesity effects in diet-induced obese mice." *Biochimica et Biophysica Acta (BBA)-Molecular and Cell Biology of Lipids* 1761, no. 7 (2006): 736-744.

132. Korhonen, Hannu, Anne Pihlanto-Leppäla, Pirjo Rantamäki, and Tuomo Tupasela. "Impact of processing on bioactive proteins and peptides." *Trends in Food Science & Technology* 9, no. 8 (1998): 307-319.

133. Kim, Sung-Eon, Young-Hun Kim, Hyungjae Lee, Dae-Ok Kim, and Hae-Yeong Kim. "Probiotic properties of lactic acid bacteria isolated from Mukeunji, a long-term ripened kimchi." *Food Science and Biotechnology* 21, no. 4 (2012): 1135-1140.

134. Knorr, Dietrich. "Technology aspects related to microorganisms in functional foods." *Trends in food science & technology* 9, no. 8 (1998): 295-306.

135. Aida, F. M. N. A., M. Shuhaimi, M. Yazid, and A. G. Maaruf. "Mushroom as a potential source of prebiotics: a review." *Trends in food science & technology* 20, no. 11 (2009): 567-575.

136. Hsieh, K-Y., C-I. Hsu, J-Y. Lin, C-C. Tsai, and R-H. Lin. "Oral administration of an edible-mushroom-derived protein inhibits the development of food-allergic reactions in mice." *Clinical & Experimental Allergy* 33, no. 11 (2003): 1595-1602.

137. 136.Liu, Yi-Hsia, Mei-Chen Kao, Yih-Loong Lai, and Jaw-Ji Tsai. "Efficacy of local nasal immunotherapy for Dp2-induced airway inflammation in mice: using Dp2 peptide and fungal immunomodulatory peptide." *Journal of allergy and clinical immunology* 112, no. 2 (2003): 301-310.

138. Fukushima, Michihiro, Masuo Nakano, Yasuko Morii, Tetsu

Ohashi, Yukiko Fujiwara, and Kei Sonoyama. "Hepatic LDL receptor mRNA in rats is increased by dietary mushroom (Agaricus bisporus) fiber and sugar beet fiber." *The Journal of nutrition* 130, no. 9 (2000): 2151-2156.

139. Handayani, D., J. Chen, Barbara J. Meyer, and Xu-Feng Huang. "Dietary Shiitake mushroom (Lentinus edodes) prevents fat deposition and lowers triglyceride in rats fed a high-fat diet." *Journal of obesity* 2011 (2011).

140. Urbain, Paul, Fabian Singler, Gabriele Ihorst, Hans-Konrad Biesalski, and Hartmut Bertz. "Bioavailability of vitamin D2 from UV-B-irradiated button mushrooms in healthy adults deficient in serum 25-hydroxyvitamin D: a randomized controlled trial." *European journal of clinical nutrition* 65, no. 8 (2011): 965-971.

141. Shimizu, Chikako, Makoto Kihara, Seiichiro Aoe, Shigeki Araki, Kazutoshi Ito, Katsuhiro Hayashi, Junji Watari, Yukikuni Sakata, and Sachie Ikegami. "Effect of high β-glucan barley on serum cholesterol concentrations and visceral fat area in Japanese men—a randomized, double-blinded, placebocontrolled trial." *Plant foods for human nutrition* 63, no. 1 (2008): 21-25.

142. Handayani, D., J. Chen, Barbara J. Meyer, and Xu-Feng Huang. "Dietary Shiitake mushroom (Lentinus edodes) prevents fat deposition and lowers triglyceride in rats fed a high-fat diet." *Journal of obesity* 2011 (2011).

143. Kim, Yea-Woon, Ki-Hoon Kim, Hyun-Ju Choi, and Dong-Seok Lee. "Anti-diabetic activity of β-glucans and their enzymatically hydrolyzed oligosaccharides from Agaricus blazei." *Biotechnology letters* 27, no. 7 (2005): 483-487.

144. James, Steven R. "Hominid use of fire in the Lower and Middle Pleistocene." *Current Anthropology* 30, no. 1 (1989): 1-26.

145. Schiller, Meinhard, Thomas Brzoska, Markus Böhm, Dieter Metze, Thomas E. Scholzen, André Rougier, and Thomas A. Luger. "Solar-simulated ultraviolet radiationinduced upregulation of the melanocortin-1 receptor, proopiomelanocortin, and α-melanocyte-stimulating hormone in human epidermis in vivo." *Journal of investigative dermatology* 122, no. 2 (2004): 468-476.

146. MacNeil, Douglas J., Andrew D. Howard, Xiaoming Guan, Tung M. Fong, Ravi P. Nargund, Maria A. Bednarek, Mark T. Goulet et al. "The role of melanocortins in body weight regulation: opportunities for the treatment of obesity." *European journal of pharmacology* 450, no. 1 (2002): 93-109.

147. Catania, Anna. "Neuroprotective actions of melanocortins: a therapeutic opportunity." *Trends in neurosciences* 31, no. 7 (2008): 353-360.

148. Cragnolini, Andrea Beatríz, Helgi Birgir Schiöth, and Teresa Nieves Scimonelli. "Anxiety-like behavior induced by IL1β is modulated by α-MSH through central melanocortin-4 receptors." *Peptides* 27, no. 6 (2006): 1451-1456.

149. Lasaga, Mercedes, Luciano Debeljuk, Daniela Durand, Teresa N. Scimonelli, and Carla Caruso. "Role of α-melanocyte stimulating hormone and melanocortin 4 receptor in brain inflammation." *Peptides* 29, no. 10 (2008): 1825-1835.

150. 149.Hadley, Mac E. "Discovery that a melanocortin regulates sexual functions in male and female humans." *Peptides* 26, no. 10 (2005): 1687-1689.

151. Golombek, Diego A., Paul Pévet, and Daniel P. Cardinali. "Melatonin effects on behavior: possible mediation by the central GABAergic system." *Neuroscience & Biobehavioral Reviews* 20, no. 3 (1996): 403-412.

152. BARTNESS, TIMOTHY J., and GEORGE N. WADE. "Photoperiodic Control of Body Weight and Energy Metabolism in Syrian Hamsters (Mesocricetus auratus): Role of Pineal Gland, Melatonin, Gonads, and Diet*." *Endocrinology114*, no. 2 (1984): 492-498.

153. Wolden-Hanson, T., D. R. Mitton, R. L. McCants, S. M. Yellon, C. W. Wilkinson, A. M. Matsumoto, and D. D. Rasmussen. "Daily Melatonin Administration to Middle-Aged Male Rats Suppresses Body Weight, Intraabdominal Adiposity, and Plasma Leptin and Insulin Independent of Food Intake and Total Body Fat 1." *Endocrinology* 141, no. 2 (2000): 487-497.

154. Gonzalez, Patricia Verónica, Helgi Birgir Schiöth, Mercedes Lasaga, and Teresa Nieves Scimonelli. "Memory impairment induced by IL-1β is reversed by α-MSH through central melanocortin-4 receptors." *Brain, behavior, and immunity* 23, no. 6 (2009): 817-822.

155. Gantz, Ira, and Tung M. Fong. "The melanocortin system." *American Journal of Physiology-Endocrinology And Metabolism* 284, no. 3 (2003): E468-E474.

156. Verret, Laure, Romain Goutagny, Patrice Fort, Laurène Cagnon, Denise Salvert, Lucienne Léger, Romuald Boissard, Paul Salin, Christelle Peyron, and Pierre-Hervé Luppi. "A role of melanin-concentrating hormone producing neurons in the central regulation of paradoxical sleep." *BMC neuroscience* 4, no. 1 (2003): 19.

157. Block, Gene D., and Terry L. Page. "Circadian pacemakers in the nervous system." *Annual review of neuroscience* 1, no. 1 (1978): 19-34.

158. Wehr, Thomas A. "Melatonin and seasonal rhythms." *Journal of biological rhythms* 12, no. 6 (1997): 518-527.

159. Xie, Y.J., Yang, D.H., Zhan, H.S., Xie, G.R.. "The Clinical Study of Manipulative Therapy on Simple Obesity: a Report of 106 Cases." *Chinese Manipulation & Qi Gong Therapy* 18 (2002): 5

160. Wu, J.W.. "Clinical Report of Treating 9198 Cases of Obesity with Tui Na Along the Channels." *Chinese Journal of Aesthetic Medicine* 8 (1999): 86-87

161. Di Lorenzo, L., G. De Pergola, C. Zocchetti, N. L'abbate, A. Basso, N. Pannacciulli, M. Cignarelli, R. Giorgino, and L. Soleo. "Effect of shift work on body mass index: results of a study performed in 319 glucose-tolerant men working in a Southern Italian industry." *International journal of obesity* 27, no. 11 (2003): 1353-1358.

162. Mohawk, Jennifer A., Carla B. Green, and Joseph S. Takahashi. "Central and peripheral circadian clocks in mammals." *Annual review of neuroscience* 35 (2012): 445.

163. Glossop, Nicholas RJ, and Paul E. Hardin. "Central and peripheral circadian oscillator mechanisms in flies and mammals." *Journal of cell science* 115, no. 17 (2002): 33693377.

164. 163.Gross, Liza. "Central and Peripheral Signals Set the Circadian Liver Clock."*PLoS biology* 5, no. 2 (2007): e50.

165. Wren, A. M., L. J. Seal, M. A. Cohen, A. E. Brynes, G. S. Frost, K. G. Murphy, W. S. Dhillo, M. A. Ghatei, and S. R. Bloom. "Ghrelin enhances appetite and increases food intake in humans." *Journal of Clinical Endocrinology & Metabolism* 86, no. 12 (2001): 5992-5992.

166. Ahima, Rexford S., Daniel Prabakaran, Christos Mantzoros, Daqing Qu, Bradford Lowell, Eleftheria Maratos-Flier, and Jeffrey S. Flier. "Role of leptin in the neuroendocrine response to fasting." (1996): 250-252.

167. Banks, William A., Christopher R. DiPalma, and Catherine L. Farrell. "Impaired transport of leptin across the blood-brain barrier in obesity☆." *Peptides* 20, no. 11 (1999): 1341-1345.

168. DING, Xing, ZHAN, Zhen. "Advances in studies on intervention effect of Chinese materia medica on blood-brain barrier." *Chinese Traditional and Herbal Drugs* 37, No. 10 (2006): 1-3.

169. Melnyk, A. N. N. A., M. E. Harper, and J. E. A. N. Himms-Hagen. "Raising at thermoneutrality prevents obesity and hyperphagia in BAT-ablated transgenic mice." *American Journal of Physiology-Regulatory, Integrative and Comparative Physiology* 272, no. 4 (1997): R1088-R1093.

170. Melnyk, Anna, and Jean Himms-Hagen. "Temperature-dependent feeding: lack of role for leptin and defect in brown adipose tissue-ablated obese mice."*American Journal of Physiology-Regulatory, Integrative and Comparative Physiology* 274, no. 4 (1998): R1131-R1135.

171. 170.Mundinger, Thomas O., David E. Cummings, and Gerald J. Taborsky Jr. "Direct stimulation of ghrelin secretion by sympathetic nerves." Endocrinology 147, no. 6 (2006): 2893-2901.

172. Sui, Y., H. L. Zhao, V. C. W. Wong, N. Brown, X. L. Li, A. K. L. Kwan, H. L. W. Hui, E. T. C. Ziea, and J. C. N. Chan. "A systematic review on use of Chinese medicine and acupuncture for treatment of obesity." *Obesity Reviews* 13, no. 5 (2012): 409-430.

173. Xie, Wei, Ling-hui Xia, Jun Fang, Hong-xia CHEN, and Wen-ning WEI. "Effect of ginsenoside Rb1 on busulfan-induced production of NO and expression of transforming growth factor beta-1 in human endothelial cells and its significance."

Chinese Journal of Hospital Pharmacy 27, no. 9 (2007): 1225.

174. Friedl, Roswitha, Thomas Moeslinger, Brigitte Kopp, and Paul Gerhard Spieckermann. "Stimulation of nitric oxide synthesis by the aqueous extract of Panax ginseng root in RAW 264.7 cells." *British journal of pharmacology* 134, no. 8 (2001): 16631670.

175. Meng, Liqiang, Lei Qu, Jiawei Tang, Shao-Qing Cai, Haiyan Wang, and Xiaomei Li. " A combination of Chinese herbs, Astragalus membranaceus var. mongholicus and Angelica sinensis, enhanced nitric oxide production in obstructed rat kidney." *Vascular pharmacology* 47, no. 2 (2007): 174-183.

176. Fang, Jian-Guo, Yun-Hai Liu, Wen-Qing Wang, Wei Xie, Shu-xian Fang, and Hong-Gang Han. "The anti-endotoxic effect of o-aminobenzoic acid from Radix Isatidis." *Acta Pharmacologica Sinica* 26, no. 5 (2005).

177. Gromicko N, Hazards CP. http://www.nachi.org/compost-pile-hazards.htm, accessed on April 26th, 2013.

178. 177.DING, Guo-yu, and Guo-xiang SUN. "Digitized HPLC fingerprints of Xiaoyao Wan [J]." *Central South Pharmacy* 3 (2011): 019.

179. Lee, Kun Yeong, and Young Jin Jeon. "Macrophage activation by polysaccharide isolated from Astragalus membranaceus." *International Immunopharmacology* 5, no. 7 (2005): 12251233.

180. Song-liu, Nie, Xu Xian-xiang, and Xia Lun-zhu. "Effect of total saponins of Codonopsis on blood lipid and nitric oxide level in experimental hyperlipemia rats." *Journal of Anhui TCM College 21*, no. 4 (2002): 40-41.

181. Jiong-ran, C. H. E. N., H. U. Ting-jun, Fu-sheng CHENG, M. E. N. G. Ju-cheng, and G. A. O. Fang. "Effect of Potentilla anserine polysaccharide on proliferation of splenic lymphocytes

and production of nitric oxide in mice [J]." *Chinese Journal of Veterinary Science and Technology* 9 (2005): 014.

182. Gardiner, Sheila M., Alix M. Compton, Terence Bennett, R. M. Palmer, and Salvador Moncada. "Control of regional blood flow by endothelium-derived nitric oxide." *Hypertension* 15, no. 5 (1990): 486-492.

183. Victoria M., Najibi, Soheil, Palacino, James J., Pagano, Patrick J., and Cohen, Richard A. "Nitric oxide directly activates calcium-dependent potassium channels in vascular smooth muscle." *Nature* 368 (1994): 850-853.

184. Bogdan, Christian. "Nitric oxide and the immune response." *Nature immunology* 2, no. 10 (2001): 907-916.

185. 184.Taylor Robinson, Andrew W., Foo Y. Liew, Alison Severn, Damo Xu, Stephen J. McSorley, Paul Garside, Julio Padron, and R. Stephen Phillips. "Regulation of the immune response by nitric oxide differentially produced by T helper type 1 and T helper type 2 cells." *European journal of immunology* 24, no. 4 (1994): 980-984.

186. Nisoli, Enzo, Emilio Clementi, Clara Paolucci, Valeria Cozzi, Cristina Tonello, Clara Sciorati, Renata Bracale et al. "Mitochondrial biogenesis in mammals: the role of endogenous nitric oxide." *Science* 299, no. 5608 (2003): 896-899.

187. Moncada, S., and E. A. Higgs. "The discovery of nitric oxide and its role in vascular biology." British journal of pharmacology 147, no. S1 (2006): S193-S201.

188. Jobgen, Wenjuan Shi, Susan K. Fried, Wenjiang J. Fu, Cynthia J. Meininger, and Guoyao Wu. "Regulatory role for the arginine–nitric oxide pathway in metabolism of energy substrates." *The Journal of nutritional biochemistry* 17, no. 9 (2006): 571-588.

189. LI, Peng-fei, Ming-sheng GUO, Da-you SHI, Nian LIU, and Zhao-xin TANG. "Accommodation of Nitric Oxide on Mitochondria Signal." *Progress in Veterinary Medicine* 10 (2010): 027.

190. Ma, Sheng-Xing. "Enhanced nitric oxide concentrations and expression of nitric oxide synthase in acupuncture points/ meridians." *The Journal of Alternative & Complementary Medicine* 9, no. 2 (2003): 207-215.

191. Tsuchiya, Masahiko, Eisuke F. Sato, Masayasu Inoue, and Akira Asada. "Acupuncture enhances generation of nitric oxide and increases local circulation." *Anesthesia & Analgesia* 104, no. 2 (2007): 301-307.

192. 191.Zhang, Yuan, Zhi-Han Tang, Zhong Ren, Shun-Lin Qu, Mi-Hua Liu, Lu-Shan Liu, and Zhi-Sheng Jiang. "Hydrogen Sulfide, the Next Potent Preventive and Therapeutic Agent in Aging and Age-Associated Diseases." *Molecular and cellular biology* 33, no. 6 (2013): 1104-1113.

193. Wang, Rui. "The gasotransmitter role of hydrogen sulfide." *Antioxidants and redox signaling* 5, no. 4 (2003): 493-501.

194. Mustafa, Asif K., Moataz M. Gadalla, and Solomon H. Snyder. "Signaling by gasotransmitters." *Science signaling* 2, no. 68 (2009): re2.

195. Olson, Kenneth R., and John A. Donald. " Nervous control of circulation–The role of gasotransmitters, NO, CO, and H2S." *Acta histochemica* 111, no. 3 (2009): 244-256.

196. Moncada, S., and E. A. Higgs. "The discovery of nitric oxide and its role in vascular biology." *British journal of pharmacology* 147, no. S1 (2006): S193-S201.

197. Barnes, Peter J., and F. Y. Liew. "Nitric oxide and asthmatic

inflammation." *Immunology today* 16, no. 3 (1995): 128-130.

198. Kaur, Harparkash, and Barry Halliwell. "Evidence for nitric oxide-mediated oxidative damage in chronic inflammation nitrotyrosine in serum and synovial fluid from rheumatoid patients." *FEBS letters* 350, no. 1 (1994): 9-12.

199. Noronha, Brian T., Jian-Mei Li, Stephen B. Wheatcroft, Ajay M. Shah, and Mark T. Kearney. "Inducible nitric oxide synthase has divergent effects on vascular and metabolic function in obesity." *Diabetes* 54, no. 4 (2005): 1082-1089.

200. Olopade, Christopher O., James A. Christon, Mohamed Zakkar, William I. Swedler, Israel Rubinstein, Chi-wei Hua, and Peter A. Scheff. "Exhaled pentane and nitric oxide levels in patients with obstructive sleep apnea." *CHEST Journal* 111, no. 6 (1997): 1500-1504.

201. 200.Lavie, Lena, Aya Hefetz, Rafael Luboshitzky, and Peretz Lavie. "Plasma levels of nitric oxide and L-arginine in sleep apnea patients." *Journal of Molecular Neuroscience* 21, no. 1 (2003): 57-63.

202. ZHANG, Sen, Zhi-zhong PAN, and Hua-shan LI. "Garlic oil stimulates murine Kupffer cell to produce nitrogen monoxide in vitro." *Immunological Journal* 2 (2004): 023.

203. LI, Y. F., and LAI, Y. "Progress on Study of Clinical Application of Allicin." Journal of Chengdu Medical College 2 (2009): 019.

204. Duh, Pin-Der, Wen Jye Yen, Pin-Chan Du, and Gow-Chin Yen. "Antioxidant activity of mung bean hulls." *Journal of the American Oil Chemists' Society* 74, no. 9 (1997): 1059-1063.

205. Wu, Shu-Jing, and Lean-Teik Ng. "Antioxidant and free radical scavenging activities of wild bitter melon (Momordica charantia

Linn. var. abbreviata Ser.) in Taiwan." *LWT-Food Science and Technology* 41, no. 2 (2008): 323-330.

206. Takahashi, Toku. "Pathophysiological significance of neuronal nitric oxide synthase in the gastrointestinal tract." *Journal of gastroenterology* 38, no. 5 (2003): 421-430.

207. Vanderwinden, Jean-Marie. "Role of nitric oxide in gastrointestinal function and disease." *Acta gastro-enterologica Belgica* 57, no. 3-4 (1993): 224-229.

208. Ellis, D.Z., Sweadner, K.J.. "NO regulation of Na,K-ATPase: nitric oxide regulation of the Na,K-ATPase in physiological and pathological states." *Annals of the New York Academy of Sciences* 986 (2003): 534-535

209. Kang, D. G., J. W. Kim, and J. Lee. "Effects of nitric oxide synthesis inhibition on the Na, K-ATPase activity in the kidney." *Pharmacological Research* 41, no. 1 (2000): 121-125.

210. 209.Whiteman, M., K. M. Gooding, J. L. Whatmore, C. I. Ball, D. Mawson, K. Skinner, J. E. Tooke, and A. C. Shore. "Adiposity is a major determinant of plasma levels of the novel vasodilator hydrogen sulphide." *Diabetologia* 53, no. 8 (2010): 1722-1726.

211. Kimura, Hideo. "Hydrogen sulfide: its production and functions." *Experimental physiology* 96, no. 9 (2011): 833-835.

212. Wang, Peipei, Gensheng Zhang, Taddese Wondimu, Brian Ross, and Rui Wang. "Hydrogen sulfide and asthma." *Experimental physiology* 96, no. 9 (2011): 847-852.

213. Dorfer, L., M. Moser, F. Bahr, K. Spindler, E. Egarter-Vigl, S. Giullen, G. Dohr, and T. Kenner. "A medical report from the stone age?." *The Lancet* 354, no. 9183 (1999): 1023-1025.

214. Kasparek, Michael S., David R. Linden, Martin E. Kreis, and

Michael G. Sarr. "Gasotransmitters in the gastrointestinal tract." *Surgery* 143, no. 4 (2008): 455.

215. Laroux, F. Stephen, David J. Lefer, Shigeyuki Kawachi, Rosario Scalia, Adam S. Cockrell, Laura Gray, Henri Van der Heyde, Jason M. Hoffman, and Matthew B. Grisham. "Role of nitric oxide in the regulation of acute and chronic inflammation." *Antioxidants and Redox Signaling* 2, no. 3 (2000): 391-396.

216. Laroux, F. Stephen, David J. Lefer, Shigeyuki Kawachi, Rosario Scalia, Adam S. Cockrell, Laura Gray, Henri Van der Heyde, Jason M. Hoffman, and Matthew B. Grisham. "Role of nitric oxide in the regulation of acute and chronic inflammation." *Antioxidants and Redox Signaling* 2, no. 3 (2000): 391-396.

217. Weiss, J. Woodrow, Yuzhen Liu, Xianghong Li, and En-sheng Ji. "Nitric oxide and obstructive sleep apnea." *Respiratory physiology & neurobiology* 184, no. 2 (2012): 192-196.

218. 217.Frühbeck, Gema, and Javier Gómez-Ambrosi. "Modulation of the leptin-induced white adipose tissue lipolysis by nitric oxide." *Cellular signalling* 13, no. 11 (2001): 827-833.

219. Moncada, Salvador. "Nitric oxide: discovery and impact on clinical medicine." *Journal of the Royal Society of Medicine* 92, no. 4 (1999): 164.

220. Moncada, S., and E. A. Higgs. "Endogenous nitric oxide: physiology, pathology and clinical relevance." *European journal of clinical investigation* 21, no. 4 (1991): 361-374.

221. Ekblad, E., P. Alm, and F. Sundler. "Distribution, origin and projections of nitric oxide synthase-containing neurons in gut and pancreas." *Neuroscience* 63, no. 1 (1994): 233-248.

222. Sweeney, Gary, and Amira Klip. "Regulation of the Na+/K+-ATPase by insulin: why and how?." In *Insulin Action,*

pp. 121

223. Springer US, 1998. 222.Iannello, Silvia, Paolina Milazzo, and Francesco Belfiore. "Animal and human tissue Na, K-ATPase in obesity and diabetes: a new proposed enzyme regulation." *The American journal of the medical sciences* 333, no. 1 (2007): 1-9.

224. Geering, Käthi. "Functional roles of Na, K-ATPase subunits." *Current opinion in nephrology and hypertension* 17, no. 5 (2008): 526-532.

225. Zhu, Xiao-Yan, Hang Gu, and Xin Ni. "Hydrogen sulfide in the endocrine and reproductive systems." (2011): 75-82.

226. Fred Hutchinson Cancer Research Center. "Could Hydrogen Sulfide Hold The Key To A Long Life?." ScienceDaily. www.sciencedaily.com/releases/2007/12/071203190614.htm (accessed February 28, 2014).

227. 226.Perna, Alessandra F., and Diego Ingrosso. "Low hydrogen sulphide and chronic kidney disease: a dangerous liaison." *Nephrology Dialysis Transplantation* 27, no. 2 (2012): 486-493.

228. Mustafa, Asif K., Moataz M. Gadalla, and Solomon H. Snyder. "Signaling by gasotransmitters." *Science signaling* 2, no. 68 (2009): re2.

229. Lee, Soo Jae, Byung-Cheon Lee, Chang Hoon Nam, Won-Chul Lee, Seong-Uk Jhang, Hyung Soon Park, and Kwang-Sup Soh. "Proteomic analysis for tissues and liquid from Bonghan ducts on rabbit intestinal surfaces." *Journal of Acupuncture and Meridian Studies* 1, no. 2 (2008): 97-109.

230. Lee, Byung-Cheon, Ho-Sung Lee, and Dae-In Kang. "Growth of microgranules into cell-like structures in fertilized chicken eggs: hypothesis for a mitosis-free alternative pathway." *Journal of acupuncture and meridian studies* 5, no. 4 (2012): 183-189.

231. Shin, Hak-Soo, Hyeon-Min Johng, Byung-Cheon Lee, Sung-Il Cho, Kyung-Soon Soh, Ku-Youn Baik, Jung-Sun Yoo, and Kwang-Sup Soh. "Feulgen reaction study of novel threadlike structures (Bonghan ducts) on the surfaces of mammalian organs." *The Anatomical Record Part B: The New Anatomist* 284, no. 1 (2005): 35-40.

232. Lee, Byung-Cheon, Jung Sun Yoo, Vyacheslav Ogay, Ki Woo Kim, Harald Dobberstein, Kwang-Sup Soh, and Byung-Soo Chang. "Electron microscopic study of novel threadlike structures on the surfaces of mammalian organs." *Microscopy Research and Technique* 70, no. 1 (2007): 34-43.

233. Sung, Baeckkyoung, Min Su Kim, Byung-Cheon Lee, Jung Sun Yoo, Sang-Hee Lee, Youn-Joong Kim, Ki-Woo Kim, and Kwang-Sup Soh. "Measurement of flow speed in the channels of novel threadlike structures on the surfaces of mammalian organs." *Naturwissenschaften* 95, no. 2 (2008): 117-124.

234. 233.Yoo, Jung Sun, Min Su Kim, Baeckkyoung Sung, Byung-Cheon Lee, Kwang-Sup Soh, Sang-Hee Lee, Youn-Joong Kim, and Harald Dobberstein. "Cribriform structure with channels in the acupuncture meridian-like system on the organ surfaces of rabbits." *ACUPUNCTURE & ELECTRO-THERAPEUTICS RESEARCH* 33, no. 1-2 (2008): 44-46.

235. Lee, Changhoon, Seung-Kwon Seol, Byung-Cheon Lee, Young-Kwon Hong, Jung-Ho Je, and Kwang-Sup Soh. "Alcian blue staining method to visualize Bonghan threads inside large caliber lymphatic vessels and X-ray microtomography to reveal their microchannels." *Lymphatic Research and Biology* 4, no. 4 (2006): 181-190.

236. Kwon, Joonhyung, Ku Youn Baik, Byung-Cheon Lee,

Kwang-Sup Soh, Nam Joo Lee, and Chi Jung Kang. "Scanning probe microscopy study of microcells from the organ surface Bonghan corpuscle." *Applied physics letters* 90, no. 17 (2007): 173903.

237. Yoo, Jung Sun, Hyeon-Min Johng, Tae-Jong Yoon, Hak-Soo Shin, Byung-Cheon Lee, Changhoon Lee, Byung Soo Ahn, Dae-In Kang, Jin-Kyu Lee, and Kwang-Sup Soh. "< i> In vivo</i> fluorescence imaging of threadlike tissues (Bonghan ducts) inside lymphatic vessels with nanoparticles." *Current Applied Physics* 7, no. 4 (2007): 342-348.

238. Lee, Byung-Cheon, Vyacheslav Ogay, Ki Woo Kim, Yuwon Lee, Jin-Kyu Lee, and Kwang-Sup Soh. "Acupuncture muscle channel in the subcutaneous layer of rat skin." *Journal of acupuncture and meridian studies* 1, no. 1 (2008): 13-19.

239. Soh, K. S., S. Hong, J. Y. Hong, B. C. Lee, and J. S. Yoo. "Immunohistochemical characterization of intravascular Bonghan duct." *Microcirculation* 13 (2006): 166.

240. Kim, M. S., J. Y. Hong, S. Hong, B. C. Lee, C. H. Nam, H. J. Woo, D. I. Kang, and K. S. Soh. "Bong-Han corpuscles as possible stem cell niches on the organ-surfaces." *J Kor Pharmacopunct Inst* 11 (2008): 5-12.

241. Lee, Soo Jae, Byung-Cheon Lee, Chang Hoon Nam, Won-Chul Lee, Seong-Uk Jhang, Hyung Soon Park, and Kwang-Sup Soh. "Proteomic analysis for tissues and liquid from Bonghan ducts on rabbit intestinal surfaces." *Journal of Acupuncture and Meridian Studies* 1, no. 2 (2008): 97-109.

242. Kim, Jungdae, Vyacheslav Ogay, Byung-Cheon Lee, Min-Su Kim, Inbin Lim, Hee-Jong Woo, Hi-Joon Park, Jan Kehr, and Kwang-Sup Soh. "Catecholamine-producing novel endocrine organ: Bonghan system." *Medical Acupuncture* 20, no. 2 (2008):

97-102.

243. Ogay, Vyacheslav, Min Su Kim, Hyo Jun Seok, Cheon Joo Choi, and Kwang-Sup Soh. "Catecholamine-storing cells at acupuncture points of rabbits." *Journal of acupuncture and meridian studies* 1, no. 2 (2008): 83-90.

244. Park, S.H., Lee, B.C., Choi, C.J., Soh, K.S., Choi, J.H., Lee, S.Y., and Ryu, P.D.. "Bioelectrical study of Bonghan Corpuscles on Organ Surfaces in Rat." *Journal of Korean Physical Society* 55, (2009): 688-693.

245. Kim, B.H.. "On the Kyungrak System." DPRK: Foreign Languages Publishing House Vol. 108 (1964): 1-38.

246. Kim, B. H.. "Sanal theory." J Acad Med Sci DPR Korea 168 (1965): 5-38.

247. Kim, B. H.. "Sanal and hematopoiesis." *J Jo Sun Med* 108 (1965): 1-6.

248. Kim, B.H.. "On the Kyungrak System." *J Acad Med Sci DPR Korea* 90 (1963): 1-41.

249. 248.Soh, K.S.. "Bonghan Duct and Acupuncture Meridian as Optical Channel of Biophoton." *Journal of the Korean Physical Society* 45 (2004): 1196–1198.

250. Bennett Davis (23 February 2002). Body Talk. Kobayashi Biophoton Lab. http://www.tohtech.ac.jp/%7Eelecs/ca/kobayashilab_hp/NewScientistE.html. Accessed on May 7th, 2013.

251. Kaznacheev, V. P., and L. I. Mikhailova. "Ultraweak radiations in intercellular interactions. Novosibirsk." *Science* (1981).

252. Cifra, Michal, Jeremy Z. Fields, and Ashkan Farhadi. "Electromagnetic cellular interactions." *Progress in biophysics and molecular biology* 105, no. 3 (2011): 223-246.

253. Vigh, B., M. J. Manzano, A. Zadori, C. L. Frank, A. Lukats, P. Rohlich, A. Szel, and C. David. "Nonvisual photoreceptors of the deep brain, pineal organs and retina." *Histology and histopathology* 17, no. 2 (2002): 555-590.

254. Schlebusch, Klaus-Peter, Walburg Maric-Oehler, and Fritz-Albert Popp. "Biophotonics in the infrared spectral range reveal acupuncture meridian structure of the body." *Journal of Alternative & Complementary Medicine* 11, no. 1 (2005): 171-173.

255. Rahnama, Majid, Jack A. Tuszynski, Istvan Bokkon, Michal Cifra, Peyman Sardar, and Vahid Salari. "Emission of mitochondrial biophotons and their effect on electrical activity of membrane via microtubules." *Journal of integrative neuroscience* 10, no. 01 (2011): 65-88.

256. George, E. "Intra-articular hyaluronan treatment for osteoarthritis." *Annals of the rheumatic diseases* 57, no. 11 (1998): 637-640.

257. 256.Grass, F., Herbert Klima, and S. Kasper. "Biophotons, microtubules and CNS, is our brain a "Holographic computer"?." *Medical hypotheses* 62, no. 2 (2004): 169-172.

258. Devaraj, Balasigamani, Masashi Usa, and Humio Inaba. "Biophotons: ultraweak light emission from living systems." *Current Opinion in Solid State and Materials Science* 2, no. 2 (1997): 188-193.

259. Sun, Yan, Chao Wang, and Jiapei Dai. "Biophotons as neural communication signals demonstrated by in situ biophoton autography." *Photochemical & Photobiological Sciences* 9, no. 3 (2010): 315-322.

260. Bk, S., M. S. Kim, V. Ogay, D. I. Kang, and K. S. Soh. "Intradermal Alcian-blue injection method to trace acupuncture meridians." *J Pharmacopunct* 11, no. 2 (2008): 5-12.

261. Fraser, J. R. E., T. C. Laurent, and U. B. G. Laurent. "Hyaluronan: its nature, distribution, functions and turnover." *Journal of internal medicine* 242, no. 1 (1997): 27-33.

262. Chen, WY John, and Giovanni Abatangelo. "Functions of hyaluronan in wound repair." *Wound Repair and Regeneration* 7, no. 2 (1999): 79-89.

263. Reichmanis, Maria, Andrew A. Marino, and Robert O. Becker. "Electrical correlates of acupuncture points." *IEEE Trans Biomed Eng* 22, no. 6 (1975): 533-535.

264. Wu, C.X., Cheng, X.M., Ding, H., Wei, X.B., Sun, X., Han, M., Song, Y.. "Effects of active ingredients in fresh ginger on levels of blood lipids and nitric oxide in rats with hyperlipidemia." *Chinese Herbal Medicines* 37 (2006): 92-94.

265. Busch, Angela J., et al. "Exercise for fibromyalgia: a systematic review." *The Journal of rheumatology* 35.6 (2008): 1130-1144.

266. Shen, Y.J.. "Pharmacology of Chinese Medicine." Shanghai Science and Technology Press. Shanghai, China: 2001

267. 265.Ohsugi, Mizue, Wenzhe Fan, Koji Hase, Quanbo Xiong, Yasuhiro Tezuka, Katsuko Komatsu, Tsuneo Namba, Tomohiro Saitoh, Kenji Tazawa, and Shigetoshi Kadota. "Active-oxygen scavenging activity of traditional nourishing-tonic herbal medicines and active constituents of Rhodiola sacra." *Journal of ethnopharmacology* 67, no. 1 (1999): 111-119.

268. Zaohua, Zhang, Liu Jianxun, Shang Xiaohong, Yang Jinhong, Chu Jinong, and Wang Zeguang. "(Institute of Information on TCM, China Academy of Traditional Chinese Medicine, Beijing 100700)□ Yao Zhiyong, Ma Honglin, Li Qingying and Wang Yin; The Effect of Rhodiola Capsules on Oxygen Consumption of Myocardium□ and Coronary Artery Blood Flow in Dogs [J]."

CHINA JOURNAL OF CHINESE MATERIA MEDICA 2 (1998).

269. Luo, Xiu-Ju, Jun Peng, and Yuan-Jian Li. "Recent advances in the study on capsaicinoids and capsinoids." *European journal of pharmacology* 650, no. 1 (2011): 1-7.

270. de La Serre, Claire Barbier, Collin L. Ellis, Jennifer Lee, Amber L. Hartman, John C. Rutledge, and Helen E. Raybould. "Propensity to high-fat diet-induced obesity in rats is associated with changes in the gut microbiota and gut inflammation." *American Journal of Physiology-Gastrointestinal and Liver Physiology* 299, no. 2 (2010): G440.

271. Joo, Jeong In, Dong Hyun Kim, Jung-Won Choi, and Jong Won Yun. "Proteomic analysis for antiobesity potential of capsaicin on white adipose tissue in rats fed with a high fat diet." *Journal of proteome research* 9, no. 6 (2010): 2977-2987.

272. Caterina, Michael J., Mark A. Schumacher, Makoto Tominaga, Tobias A. Rosen, Jon D. Levine, and David Julius. "The capsaicin receptor: a heat-activated ion channel in the pain pathway." *Nature* 389, no. 6653 (1997): 816-824.

273. 271.Deal, Chad L., Thomas J. Schnitzer, E. Lipstein, James R. Seibold, Randall M. Stevens, Moise D. Levy, D. Albert, and F. Renold. "Treatment of arthritis with topical capsaicin: a double-blind trial." *Clinical therapeutics* 13, no. 3 (1990): 383- 395.

274. Yoshida, T., K. Yoshioka, Y. Wakabayashi, H. Nishioka, and M. Kondo. "Effects of capsaicin and isothiocyanate on thermogenesis of interscapular brown adipose tissue in rats." *Journal of nutritional science and vitaminology* 34, no. 6 (1988): 587-594.

275. Kong, Dong, Qingchun Tong, Chianping Ye, Shuichi Koda, Patrick M. Fuller, Michael J. Krashes, Linh Vong, Russell S. Ray,

David P. Olson, and Bradford B. Lowell. "GABAergic RIP-Cre neurons in the arcuate nucleus selectively regulate energy expenditure." *Cell* 151, no. 3 (2012): 645-657.

276. Jahnke, Roger, et al. "A comprehensive review of health benefits of qigong and tai chi." *American Journal of Health Promotion* 24.6 (2010): e1-e25.

277. Velićanski, Aleksandra S., Dragoljub D. Cvetković, Siniša L. Markov, Vesna T. Tumbas, and Slađana M. Savatović. "Antimicrobial and antioxidant activity of lemon balm Kombucha." *Acta periodica technologica* 38 (2007): 165-172.

278. Cetojevic-Simin, D. D., G. M. Bogdanovic, D. D. Cvetkovic, and A. S. Velicanski. "Antiproliferative and antimicrobial activity of traditional Kombucha and Satureja montana L. Kombucha." *Journal of BU ON.: official journal of the Balkan Union of Oncology* 13, no. 3 (2007): 395-401.

279. University of Alabama at Birmingham. "Garlic Boosts Hydrogen Sulfide To Relax Arteries." ScienceDaily. www.sciencedaily. com/releases/2007/10/071016131534.htm (accessed March 4, 2014).

280. Fan, Yi-Fei, Zhi-Wu Chen, Yan Guo, Qi-Hai Wang, and Biao Song. "Cellular mechanisms underlying Hyperin-induced relaxation of rat basilar artery." *Fitoterapia* 82, no. 4 (2011): 626-631.

281. Liu, Ying, Li-Ping Zou, Jun-Bao Du, and Virginia Wong. "Electro-acupuncture protects against hypoxic–ischemic brain-dama*ged immature rat via hydrogen sulfide as a possible mediator.*" *Neuroscience letters* 485, no. 1 (2010): 74-78.

282. The Peninsula College of Medicine and Dentistry. "Lower levels of 'rotten egg' gas (hydrogen sulfide) in blood linked to obesity, type 2 diabetes and poorer circulation." ScienceDaily.

www.sciencedaily.com/releases/2010/04/100427190937.htm (accessed March 4, 2014).

283. Langhorst, Jost, et al. "Efficacy and safety of meditative movement therapies in fibromyalgia syndrome: a systematic review and meta-analysis of randomized controlled trials." *Rheumatology International* 33.1 (2013): 193-207.

284. Lynch, Mary, et al. "A randomized controlled trial of qigong for fibromyalgia."*Arthritis Research and Therapy* 14.4 (2012): R178.

285. Maddali, Bongi S., et al. "Resseguier method and Qi Gong sequentially integrated in patients with fibromyalgia syndrome." *Clinical and experimental rheumatology* 30.6 Suppl 74 (2011): 51-58.

286. Whiteman, M., K. M. Gooding, J. L. Whatmore, C. I. Ball, D. Mawson, K. Skinner, J. E. Tooke, and A. C. Shore. "Adiposity is a major determinant of plasma levels of the novel vasodilator hydrogen sulphide." *Diabetologia* 53, no. 8 (2010): 1722-1726.

287. Medani, Mekki, Danielle Collins, Neil G. Docherty, Alan W. Baird, Patrick R. O'Connell, and Des C. Winter. "Emerging role of hydrogen sulfide in colonic physiology and pathophysiology." *Inflammatory bowel diseases* 17, no. 7 (2011): 1620-1625.

288. 孙大定. "辛味药的药性理论及其配伍作用初探."中国中药杂志 8 (1992): 17.

289. Jones, Kim D., and Ginevra L. Liptan. "Exercise interventions in fibromyalgia: clinical applications from the evidence." *Rheumatic Disease Clinics of North America* 35.2 (2009): 373-391.

290. SHENG, Kang-mei, and Hong-jie WANG. "Advances in Research of Chemical Constituents and Pharmacological Activites of Arillus Longan [J]." *Chinese Journal of Experimental*

Traditional Medical Formulae 5 (2010): 080.

291. 284.Jian, Chen, Lu Yongmei, and Wu Fengling. "Study on experiments and clinical application of dark plum aerosol to relieve xerostomia of postoperative patients after accepting gastrointestinal tract operation." *Chinese Nursing Research* 27 (2011): 017.

292. 王晓红, 李雅梅, and 张燕. "乌梅的临床应用." 医药导报 S1 (2003).

293. Yingfu, Zhang, Qiu Xiaoqing, and Tian Zhifeng. "Study of Dark Plum on Contractile Activity of Isolated Bladder Detrusor Muscle of Guinea Pigs [J]."*SHANXI JOURNAL OF TRADITIONAL CHINESE MEDICINE 2* (2000): 035.

294. Chen, Kevin W., et al. "A pilot study of external qigong therapy for patients with fibromyalgia." *Journal of Alternative & Complementary Medicine* 12.9 (2006): 851-856.

295. Haak, Thomas, and Berit Scott. "The effect of Qigong on fibromyalgia (FMS): a controlled randomized study." *Disability and rehabilitation* 30.8 (2008): 625-633.

296. Sephton, Sandra E., et al. "Mindfulness meditation alleviates depressive symptoms in women with fibromyalgia: results of a randomized clinical trial."*Arthritis Care & Research* 57.1 (2007): 77-85.

297. Taggart, Helen M., et al. "Effects of T'ai Chi exercise on fibromyalgia symptoms and health-related quality of life." *Orthopaedic Nursing* 22.5 (2003): 353-360.

298. Wang, Chenchen, et al. "A randomized trial of tai chi for fibromyalgia." *New England Journal of Medicine* 363.8 (2010): 743-754.

299. Zhou, Muke, et al. "A randomized trial of tai chi for

fibromyalgia." *The New England journal of medicine* 363.23 (2010): 2265-author.

300. Krawinkel, Michael B., and Gudrun B. Keding. "Bitter gourd (Momordica charantia): a dietary approach to hyperglycemia." *Nutrition reviews* 64, no. 7 (2006): 331-337.

301. F Fang, E., and T. B Ng. "Bitter gourd (Momordica charantia) is a cornucopia of health: a review of its credited antidiabetic, anti-HIV, and antitumor properties."*Current molecular medicine* 11, no. 5 (2011): 417-436.

302. Lee, Bombi, Bongjun Sur, Mijung Yeom, Insop Shim, Hyejung Lee, and Dae-Hyun Hahm. "Effect of berberine on depression- and anxiety-like behaviors and activation of the noradrenergic system induced by development of morphine dependence in rats." *The Korean Journal of Physiology & Pharmacology* 16, no. 6 (2012): 379-386.

303. Hua Lliang, Wei Xia, Linhong Yuan and Kun Wu. "Effects of celery extract on blood pressure of SHRand serum lipid of experimental hyperlipidmia rats." *China Journey of Disease Control Preview* 9, no. 2 (2005): 97-99.

304. PANG, Guang-chang, Li-qin YU, and Tian-ye MA. "Study on Causal Relationship of Foods, Rabbit Body Temperature and Immunoregulation." *Food Science* 10 (2008): 139.

305. 张斌. "中药四性理论的表述及黄连, 栀子, 干姜, 附子对正常大鼠效应的实验研究." Master's thesis, 山东中医药大学, 2008.

306. 高琳. "干姜不同有效部位对理中丸调节脾阳虚模型消化功能及能量代谢的影响." PhD diss.,北京中医药大学, 2009.

307. 秦华珍. "酸味, 涩味药药性, 化学成分, 药理作用探讨."湖南中医学院学报 18, no. 3 (1998): 64-65.

308. 于培明, 田智勇, and 陈随清. "咸味药的药性理论及其配伍探讨." 国医论坛 20, no. 1 (2005): 48-49.

309. 于培明, 田智勇, and 林桂涛. "甘味药的药性理论及其配伍探讨." 时珍国医国药16, no. 1 (2005): 77-78.

310. 廉秀云, 吴运玲, and 冯惠善. "浅谈苦味药的药性特征及其配伍作用."黑龙江中医药 1 (1991): 52-53.

311. 周典铭, and 熊轩玖. "辛味药的药性理论及其配伍作用初探."湖北中医学院学报2, no. 2 (2000): 48-49.

312. "1,458 Bacteria Species 'New to Science' Found in Our Belly Buttons"http://www.theatlantic.com/health/archive/2012/12/1-458-bacteria-species-new-to-science-found-in-our-belly-buttons/266360/(accessed April 4, 2014).

313. Sutton-Grier, Ariana E., Justin P. Wright, Bonnie M. McGill, and Curtis Richardson. "Environmental conditions influence the plant functional diversity effect on potential denitrification." *PloS one* 6, no. 2 (2011): e16584.

314. LI, Run-ping, Sheng-shan ZHU, Wei-yao WU, Yan-qu CAI, and Zhi-wei SU. "Research Progress in Chemical Composition and Pharmacological Effects of Baoji Pills." *Chinese Journal of Experimental Traditional Medical Formulae* 11 (2010): 064. (保济丸中化学成分与药理作用研究进展)

315. Dressaire, Emilie, Junius Santoso, Lisa Yamada, and Marcus Roper. "Control of fluidic environments by mushrooms." *Bulletin of the American Physical Society* 58 (2013).

316. Cao, Huijuan, JianPing Liu, and George T. Lewith. "Traditional Chinese Medicine for treatment of fibromyalgia: a systematic review of randomized controlled trials." *The Journal of Alternative and Complementary Medicine*16.4 (2010): 397-409.

317. Cao, Huijuan, et al. "Acupoint stimulation for fibromyalgia: a systematic review of randomized controlled trials." *Evidence-Based Complementary and Alternative Medicine* 2013 (2013).

318. Montana State University. "Microbes swim to hydrogen gas." ScienceDaily. www.sciencedaily.com/ releases/2013/11/131109153935.htm (accessed January 31, 2014).

319. Jastreboff, Ania M. "Oxytocin Curbs Cookie Consumption." *Science Translational Medicine* 5, no. 208 (2013): 208ec173-208ec173.

320. Kerti, Lucia, A. Veronica Witte, Angela Winkler, Ulrike Grittner, Dan Rujescu, and Agnes Flöel. "Higher glucose levels associated with lower memory and reduced hippocampal microstructure." *Neurology* 81, no. 20 (2013): 1746-1752.

321. Zhang, Yuanfen, Lil Träskman-Bendz, Shorena Janelidze, Patricia Langenberg, Ahmed Saleh, Niel Constantine, Olaoluwa Okusaga, Cecilie Bay-Richter, Lena Brundin, and Teodor T. Postolache. "Toxoplasma gondii immunoglobulin G antibodies and nonfatal suicidal self-directed violence." *J Clin Psychiatry* 73, no. 8 (2012): 1069-1076.

322. Dotta, B. T., K. S. Saroka, and Michael A. Persinger. "Increased photon emission from the head while imagining light in the dark is correlated with changes in electroencephalographic power: Support for Bókkon's biophoton hypothesis." *Neuroscience letters* 513, no. 2 (2012): 151-154.

323. Cohen, S., and F. A. Popp. "Biophoton emission of the human body." *Journal of Photochemistry and Photobiology B: Biology* 40, no. 2 (1997): 187-189.

324. Glombiewski, Julia A., et al. "Psychological treatments for

fibromyalgia: a meta-analysis." *PAIN®* 151.2 (2010): 280-295.

325. Dinan, Timothy G., and John F. Cryan. "Regulation of the stress response by the gut microbiota: implications for psychoneuroendocrinology." Psychoneuroendocrinology 37, no. 9 (2012): 1369-1378.

326. Miquel, Jaime. "An update of the oxidation-inflammation theory of aging: the involvement of the immune system in oxi-inflamm-aging." *Current pharmaceutical design* 15, no. 26 (2009): 3003-3026.

327. Pearce, Laura R., Neli Atanassova, Matthew C. Banton, Bill Bottomley, Agatha A. van der Klaauw, Jean-Pierre Revelli, Audrey Hendricks et al. "KSR2 Mutations Are Associated with Obesity, Insulin Resistance, and Impaired Cellular Fuel Oxidation." *Cell* 155, no. 4 (2013): 765-777.

328. Aguilera, Margarita, María Luján Jiménez-Pranteda, Barbara Jenko, Verónica Jiménez, and Marisa Cañadas Garre. "Pharmacogenomics and Gut Microbiota Biomarkers in Obesity." *In Omics for Personalized Medicine*, pp. 575-601. Springer India, 2013.

329. Requena, Teresa, Paul Cotter, Danit R. Shahar, Charlotte R. Kleiveland, M. Carmen Martínez-Cuesta, Carmen Peláez, and Tor Lea. "Interactions between gut microbiota, food and the obese host." *Trends in Food Science & Technology* 34, no. 1 (2013): 44-53.

330. Legler, Juliette. "An Integrated Approach to Assess the Role of Chemical Exposure in Obesity." *Obesity* 21, no. 6 (2013): 1084-1085.

331. Larsen, Lesli Hingstrup. "Obesity: Underlying Mechanisms and the Evolving Influence of Diet." *Current Nutrition Reports* 1, no. 4 (2012): 205-214.

332. Manco, Melania. "Gut microbiota and developmental programming of the brain: from evidence in behavioral endophenotypes to novel perspective in obesity."*Frontiers in cellular and infection microbiology* 2 (2012).

333. Milagro, Fermín I., M. L. Mansego, C. De Miguel, and José Alfredo Martinez. "Dietary factors, epigenetic modifications and obesity outcomes: Progresses and perspectives." *Molecular aspects of medicine* 34, no. 4 (2013): 782-812.

334. Vaahtovuo, Jussi, Eveliina Munukka, MIKA KORKEAMÄKI, Reijo Luukkainen, and Paavo Toivanen. "Fecal microbiota in early rheumatoid arthritis." *The Journal of rheumatology* 35, no. 8 (2008): 1500-1505.

335. Chisholm, Stephen T., Gitta Coaker, Brad Day, and Brian J. Staskawicz. "Host-microbe interactions: shaping the evolution of the plant immune response." *Cell* 124, no. 4 (2006): 803-814.

336. Salzman, Nita H. "Microbiota–immune system interaction: an uneasy alliance." *Current opinion in microbiology* 14, no. 1 (2011): 99-105.

337. Collins, Stephen M., Michael Surette, and Premysl Bercik. "The interplay between the intestinal microbiota and the brain." *Nature Reviews Microbiology* 10, no. 11 (2012): 735-742.

338. Zhang, Yuanfen, Lil Traskman-Bendz, Shorena Janelidze, Patricia Langenberg, Ahmed Saleh, Niel Constantine, Olaoluwa Okusaga, Cecilie Bay-Richter, Lena Brundin, and Teodor T. Postolache. "Toxoplasma gondii immunoglobulin G antibodies and nonfatal suicidal self-directed violence." *J Clin psychiatry* 73, no. 8 (2012): 1069-1076.

339. Ley, Ruth E., Peter J. Turnbaugh, Samuel Klein, and Jeffrey I. Gordon. "Microbial ecology: human gut microbes associated

with obesity." *Nature* 444, no. 7122 (2006): 1022-1023.

340. 324.Turnbaugh, Peter J., Micah Hamady, Tanya Yatsunenko, Brandi L. Cantarel, Alexis Duncan, Ruth E. Ley, Mitchell L. Sogin et al. "A core gut microbiome in obese and lean twins." *Nature* 457, no. 7228 (2009): 480-484.

341. Dressaire, Emilie, Junius Santoso, Lisa Yamada, and Marcus Roper. "Control of fluidic environments by mushrooms." *Bulletin of the American Physical Society* 58 (2013).

342. Galynker, Igor, Christie Ieronimo, Alvin Perez-Acquino, Yick Lee, and Arnold Winston. "Panic attacks with psychotic features." *The Journal of clinical psychiatry* 57, no. 9 (1996): 402-406.

343. Kim, Do-Hoon, Yoo-Sun Moon, Hee-Sung Kim, Jun-Sub Jung, Hyung-Moo Park, Hong-Won Suh, Yung-Hi Kim, and Dong-Keun Song. "Effect of Zen Meditation on serum nitric oxide activity and lipid peroxidation." *Progress in Neuro-Psychopharmacology and Biological Psychiatry* 29, no. 2 (2005): 327-331.

344. Thauer, Rudolf K. "Biochemistry of methanogenesis: a tribute to Marjory Stephenson: 1998 Marjory Stephenson Prize Lecture." *Microbiology* 144, no. 9 (1998): 2377-2406.

345. Leffler, Charles W., Helena Parfenova, Jonathan H. Jaggar, and Rui Wang. "Carbon monoxide and hydrogen sulfide: gaseous messengers in cerebrovascular circulation." *Journal of Applied Physiology* 100, no. 3 (2006): 1065-1076.

346. Pan, Xiaogui, Yi Zhang, and Sai Tao. "Effects of Tai Chi exercise on blood pressure and plasma levels of nitric oxide, carbon monoxide and hydrogen sulfide in real-world patients with essential hypertension." *Clinical and Experimental Hypertension* 0 (2014): 1-7.

347. Dhir, Ashish, and S. K. Kulkarni. "Nitric oxide and major

depression." *Nitric Oxide* 24, no. 3 (2011): 125-131.

348. 332.Sarri, Katerina O., Nikolaos E. Tzanakis, Manolis K. Linardakis, George D. Mamalakis, and Anthony G. Kafatos. "Effects of Greek Orthodox Christian Church fasting on serum lipids and obesity." *BMC Public Health* 3, no. 1 (2003): 16.

349. Sarri, Katerina O., Nikolaos E. Tzanakis, Manolis K. Linardakis, George D. Mamalakis, and Anthony G. Kafatos. "Effects of Greek Orthodox Christian Church fasting on serum lipids and obesity." *BMC Public Health* 3, no. 1 (2003): 16.

350. Chen, Yan, and Lihong Liu. "Modern methods for delivery of drugs across the blood–brain barrier." *Advanced drug delivery reviews* 64, no. 7 (2012): 640-665.

351. Hui, YANG Ling, Z. O. U. Da Jin, FENG Zheng Kang, L. U. Jin, L. I. U. Yan, and WU Wen Jun. "Effect of Radix astragali on insulin sensitivity in high-fat-fed rats [J]." *Academic Journal of Second Military Medical University* 4 (2004): 022.

352. Qian, Hao, Michael J. Azain, Mark M. Compton, Diane L. Hartzell, Gary J. Hausman, and Clifton A. Baile. "Brain administration of leptin causes deletion of adipocytes by apoptosis." *Endocrinology* 139, no. 2 (1998): 791-794.

353. de Man, Frits H., Rienk Nieuwland, Arnoud van der Laarse, Fred Romijn, Augustinus HM Smelt, Jan A. Gevers Leuven, and Augueste Sturk. "Activated platelets in patients with severe hypertriglyceridemia: effects of triglyceride-lowering therapy." *Atherosclerosis* 152, no. 2 (2000): 407-414.

354. Bansal, Sandeep, Julie E. Buring, Nader Rifai, Samia Mora, Frank M. Sacks, and Paul M. Ridker. "Fasting compared with nonfasting triglycerides and risk of cardiovascular events in women." *Jama* 298, no. 3 (2007): 309-316.

355. 339.Igna, Cornel Victor, Juhani Julkunen, and Hannu Vanhanen. "Vital exhaustion, depressive symptoms and serum triglyceride levels in high-risk middle-aged men." *Psychiatry research* 187, no. 3 (2011): 363-369.

356. Fond, Guillaume, Alexandra Macgregor, Marion Leboyer, and Andreas Michalsen. "Fasting in mood disorders: neurobiology and effectiveness. A review of the literature." *Psychiatry research* 209, no. 3 (2013): 253-258.

357. 盲人摸象 (Mang Ren Mo Xiang Blind men and an elephant) picture retrieved on March 22, 2014 from http://ziyiwondering.blogspot.com/2013/04/die-blinden-manner-und-der-elefant.html

Made in the USA
Middletown, DE
16 February 2018